Love Food and Be Slim!

Motivational Secrets for the Body You
Desire and the Success You Crave

Natasha Reddy

With a foreword by Dr Isaac Jones,
founder of designerhealthcenters.com

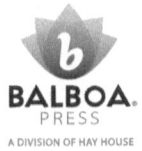

BALBOA.
PRESS

A DIVISION OF HAY HOUSE

ISBN: 978-1-4525-4593-6 (sc)
ISBN: 978-1-4525-4594-3 (e)
ISBN: 978-1-4525-4595-0 (hc)

Library of Congress Control Number: 2012901636

Balboa Press books may be ordered through booksellers or by contacting:

Balboa Press
A Division of Hay House
1663 Liberty Drive
Bloomington, IN 47403
www.balboapress.com
1-(877) 407-4847

Because of the dynamic nature of the Internet, any web addresses or links contained in this book may have changed since publication and may no longer be valid. The views expressed in this work are solely those of the author and do not necessarily reflect the views of the publisher, and the publisher hereby disclaims any responsibility for them.

The author of this book does not dispense medical advice or prescribe the use of any technique as a form of treatment for physical, emotional, or medical problems without the advice of a physician, either directly or indirectly. The intent of the author is only to offer information of a general nature to help you in your quest for emotional and spiritual well-being. In the event you use any of the information in this book for yourself, which is your constitutional right, the author and the publisher assume no responsibility for your actions.

Any people depicted in stock imagery provided by Thinkstock are models, and such images are being used for illustrative purposes only.
Certain stock imagery © Thinkstock.

Printed in the United States of America

Balboa Press rev. date:3/14/2012

I dedicate this book to my Anjali.
To me, you are beauty itself.
But always remember, my daughter,
'Beauty is not in the face; Beauty is a light in the heart.' Kahlil Gibran

'It's not the diet that counts: it's *who you have to be* to follow the diet that counts. Yet, every year millions of people look for the perfect diet to follow in order to become thin. They focus on what they have to do, rather than who they have to be. A diet will not help if your thoughts do not change.'
Robert Kiyosaki, *Rich Dad, Poor Dad 2*

Contents

Foreword

Sarah has just dropped her kids off at school on her way to meet up with some girlfriends she hasn't seen in a few months. She pulls up to the restaurant, eager to catch up on all the drama that's been going on in their lives. But she thinks to herself, 'I feel fat, I probably look fat and I sure hope that my girlfriends don't notice the 5lb I've gained since the last time I saw them.' She walks into the beautiful Ritz-like restaurant to meet her friends, and as she approaches them she sees them looking her up and down. One of her skinny friends seems to fall into a three-second trance as she stares at her waistline, before shaking herself out of it. As Sarah steps up to greet her friends with a hug, she thinks, 'They've noticed... Is it that obvious?'

The girlfriends all have their 'my life is perfect' smiley faces on and the catching up begins. As Sarah is talking, she can't help but notice how good a few of her friends look. She thinks to herself, 'I need to go on a diet. I feel fat and ugly, especially around these couple of twigs!' Seeing her skinny girlfriends is the leverage she needs to make change.

On the way home she stops by the local bookstore and looks at the hundreds of diet books on the shelf. One says, 'Lose 15 pounds in 20 days,' another says, '5-minute meals to lose 5 pounds of belly fat' and yet another says, 'The 1 step to take to lose that ugly fat once and for all.' The authors consist of PhDs, nutritionists and other alleged weight-loss experts.

Sarah picks up a baby-blue book that seems less sales-like and more down to earth. She reads it and follows the programme to a 't', and guess what happens...? She loses 10lb! She's happy, her husband is happy and she's excited at the prospect of meeting up with her girlfriends for their next get-together in a month's time.

But guess what happens then? By the time she meets up with her girlfriends again, she's gained all her weight back plus 5lb.

How could this be? Sarah was on a roll, right?

The reality is, you can eat all the right foods, but if you don't address the underlying cause of your extra weight then you won't lose weight in the long term. Period. This story of Sarah is the sad story of over 90 per cent of dieters, because 90 per cent of dieters fail.

There are more dieting books on the market now than ever before and yet people are carrying around more disease-causing, esteem-crushing fat than ever before. People go on diets to look and feel sexy again and get healthy, but what do they actually get? In the long run it's usually several more pounds around their belly. Because for the most part, diets fail to address the root cause of the problem or the reason why people get fat. So I'm going to tell you exactly what the root cause of that problem is and how this incredible book helps to address it.

I know it truly is possible to get incredible weight-loss results without dieting, because I see it every day with people who go through my online programmes. How? I get people to make the conscious decision to change their goals from 'losing weight' through a short-term diet to adopting a long-term sustainable realistic lifestyle, or what I call 'lifestyling'. When someone's 'lifestyling', they are eating healthily, thinking healthily and adopting a new identity of being slim, hence the title of this book! When you do this, you won't just look good in a bikini for one summer, but for every summer! If you're a guy, this is your fastest track to rocking that six-pack you've always wanted (and no, I'm not talking about the type that goes in the fridge). The research is conclusive: dieting is dead and lifestyling is the only way to lose weight month after month until you get to what Natasha calls your 'healthiest weight' and reveal the body of your dreams.

However, it's easier said than done. How does someone deal with the emotional baggage, self-sabotaging psychology and bad habits that keep them fat? The human condition is a complex one. We come with baggage, right? Sarah lost 10lb over 2 months and gained everything back plus some just a month later. How could she have continued to lose 10lb every 2 months (60lb a year) until she got to her ideal weight instead? How could she have done that while enjoying the process and loving the food she ate? It comes down to what Natasha Reddy has so brilliantly outlined in the pages of this book.

Losing weight and keeping the weight off have to do with changing your thinking and creating long-term sustainable health habits. If you want to lose weight in the long term, you have to address what's going on between your ears. If you want to lose weight and enjoy your life, then Natasha will walk you through the process to do so. She will soon be considered one of the top experts in weight-loss psychology today. In this book she will help you take on a new and empowering identity that will melt fat off your body. She will take you through 28 powerful keys to thinking differently that will help to address the cause of your weight challenges. Once you have your mindset right, her 10 super-strategies will inject even more weight-loss juice into your mind to solidify your success psychology. And what do you do once you've emptied and cleaned your mind and downloaded the new weight-loss software? You follow the 10 powerful food habits and learn about how to become nutritionally aware and exercise savvy! Your body will celebrate as you follow the life-changing content on these pages. Natasha then finishes the book with a 28-day food awareness plan that will reveal to you how and what to eat until eating healthily becomes a natural part of your life. What more could you ask for in a weight-loss book? If you follow what Natasha tells you, it will not only get you skinny, it will transform your life!

Welcome to the beginning of your new body and your new life!

To true health and real results,

Dr Isaac Jones
designerhealthcenters.com

Acknowledgements

This book is the fulfilment of a dream, so thanks a million to:

My family – my amazing husband and gorgeous children – for the moments I 'stole' from you to tap away. Thanks for your loving support and your unswerving patience with my being 'artistically' anti-social! To my in-laws, 'Uncle' and my 'Atta-garu', and my own parents: love you all!

My friends Judith O'Reilly, of *Wife in the North*, and Jenni O'Connor, who made me think I might be capable of writing a book too!

Penelope Trunk, of the Brazen Careerist, who pushed me over the edge into motivation.

Velile Ndebele, of London's Aqualibria hydrotherapy clinic, who forced me to think creatively.

Nick Williams, author of *Unconditional Success,* who first encouraged me by showing interest.

My amazingly inspiring entrepreneur friends Robert Webb and Daniele Poggio.

Rachel Elnaugh, whose seminars enlightened me.

The David Gold, who told me to 'go for it' (and I've got the photo to prove it!)

Lord Jeffrey Archer, who inspired 'Ruthless Discipline'!

Christopher Howard, who introduced me to the very useful concept of 'chunking'.

Indirectly to Tony Robbins, Robert and Kim Kiyosaki, Donald Trump, Richard Branson, Richard Templar, Duncan Bannatyne, Sahar Hashemi, Susie Orbach, Chris Howard, Kerwin Rae and the many, many successful luminaries whose work I envy and admire.

Especially to those who first introduced me to NLP: old friends Bobby Singh and Frank Frikker, and Masterful creator Richard Bandler, who gave me a raw insight.

Ali Campbell, my first celebrity life coach, who generously gave me time and advice and forgave me (I hope!) even when I allowed things *not* to be effortless at all!

Also, thanks and so much gratitude to a new friend and exceptionally creative genius (and interior designer), Annie Friend, who in our discussions about this book contributed so much meaningful advice.

To Ray Stevens, Olympic silver medallist, judo master and business owner, thank you for your endorsement. Your judo classes and fitness clubs are second to none!

To Lizzie Hutchins, my esteemed editor – I might be the creator, but you're the sculptor! A thousand thanks for a job very well done.

Most exceptionally, thanks to Dr Isaac and Erica Jones, pioneers of the New Health Model, who are changing the planet's health globally, one person at a time, and who have been my greatest support throughout this book, and to my teacher Steve Linder, who gave me the tools to live from the heart and to serve others. I can never express my thanks enough to you guys, whose teachings and support have been my lifeline throughout!

And lastly, thanks for divine inspiration. My gratitude is beyond words.

Introduction

This book is *not* a weight-loss manual. It's a journey to a new way of thinking – and once you buy your ticket, there's no going back!

It's my belief that anyone can lose weight and feel more confident and energetic. Excluding those with certain rare medical conditions, no one is born fat. Weight gain is a behavioural trait. It's as much to do with how we behave around food as it is to do with the food itself. It's also a lot to do with *identity* – how we see ourselves and what we believe about food. So, when you concentrate on understanding and applying the information in this book, not only will you be in the best position ever to *lose* weight but also to *gain* much more: more self-confidence, more happiness, more contentment and more fulfilment.

How to Use This Book

This is a book for people everywhere – people just like you. And the best news is, you've no need to set aside large amounts of time and money for specialist diet plans, particular ingredients, fiddly recipes or group meetings. Instead, just read the information in this book very carefully and incorporate it into your life, day by day. It really is that simple. All you have to remember is to *take action*. The more you *act* on the information you're learning, the more powerful it will be! That way you'll be increasing the likelihood of losing weight not just on a short-term basis, but for good. And by changing the way you think, you'll also be developing a mindset for success in all areas of your life!

Thinking differently is a brand new experience. It might feel a little strange at the outset, but as soon as the process is up and running, it'll feel like a breeze, as everything *suddenly just clicks*. The secret is to think it through and fit the advice in this book into your daily lifestyle, making it work for you individually.

To help you, I'm going to provide you with *Keys* to turn to open a new way of thinking. You'll discover that these address not just the symptoms of overeating but also *why* you are overeating in the first place. And before you say, 'But I *don't* overeat!', if you have excess weight, either your portions are too large, or you graze too much, or you eat too many highly-calorific foods and do too little exercise… Sound familiar?

All about *You*

So, commit to losing that excess weight, feeling better, breaking out of emotional eating patterns and becoming more confident. Commit to creating positive energy in your life, because it's all about energy. Take note – this is probably the most important thing you will ever learn!

Take pen and paper and write it down:

> *'Whatever energy I am creating in my life determines my life.'*

It's that simple. Sadness and happiness, for example, are simply forms of energy. Frustration and dissatisfaction are just energy. Feeling good is also just energy. And energy is contagious – which is why happy people make other people happy!

We all have our different brand and level of energy, which is why, like snowflakes, no two 'dieters' are ever alike. People overeat for different reasons, are built differently and have different lifestyles and metabolisms. So, you're going to create your own strategies for eating and exercise and well-being. You're going to optimize your own behaviour to meet your own needs and goals. You're going to make it all about *you*.

A Change in Mindset

Because one size does not fit all, I am not guaranteeing that *every* piece of advice in this book will suit every reader. So, choose what suits you best. But every time you make a decision, or think a thought, or feel a feeling, remember your goals, and remember you can succeed! You can succeed in this – and much more besides!

How do I know this? It's time to tell you about myself. I used to work in the City of London, in what was called a 'Big Five' firm. I was contracted out to a lot of banks. I found that watching how people behaved and what motivated them was much more exciting than the projects themselves. Then I moved to Tokyo, where I trained top executives in communication and negotiation skills.

After having my two children, I retrained as a certified Neurostrategist, a licensed Master Practitioner of Neuro-Linguistic Programming (with Richard Bandler, the founding father) and a certified hypnotherapist with the American Association of Hypnotherapy.

When I started this book, I was mulling over a couple of different titles. Then one day I was chatting with a new friend, Annie. We were talking about how sad it was that some people called food 'naughty'. After all, it's just food, isn't it? How can it possibly be 'naughty'? That's just a projection, when the *person* eating it has feelings of guilt. It's never the *food*'s fault, is it?

'Thing is, food has so many emotional associations,' said Annie. We discussed how food could be a comforter for some, a sticking plaster for others, and how some people hid behind being overweight for reasons that had nothing whatsoever to do with food. We talked about how diets didn't work long term if the behaviour underlying them didn't change. We talked about how food was inextricably bound up with *identity*. We talked about this book.

This book is about long-term change. It's not about quick fixes, menu changes or hitting the gym if you've always been a couch potato. It's about learning to work with who you are to get the results you want. It's about understanding who you are and what makes you tick – what drives your behaviour. It's about a 'shift in mindset'. That's the buzz phrase! Once you understand the strategies underlying your behaviour, you can change them. And transform your life.

It can take just a single moment of realization. Yes, it really can be that simple. Here's a testimonial from my very first client (coaching for motivation, not weight loss, but the process is the same):

> 'Natasha Reddy has a wonderful means of getting to
> the root of the problem without one even noticing, and
> within this same moment, a solution has been found.'

> J. Hay, Wimbledon, ballet dancer and teacher

And after that first transformational moment, then what? The key to success is not to 'meditate and have a bag of money fall on your head',[1] but to take *action*. You can think, dream, manifest, meditate, wish and pray all you want, but if you don't take *action*, you won't get results!

Taking action needn't be hard. In fact, it has to be simple and easy. That way, you'll enjoy it and go the stretch. Do you think a mega-successful businessman like Richard Branson or Donald Trump finds making money hard work or enjoys the process? Why do you think they're so successful? Could it be because they're *loving every minute of it*?

You too can make realizing your goals easy and enjoyable. Let's start with creating your very own special sense of responsibility to yourself. You want to do the best by yourself, don't you? I know you do, or you wouldn't have bought this book. I call this lovely sense of wanting the best for yourself 'living at cause',[2] as opposed to 'living at effect'. When you live at effect, you're a victim who thinks everyone else is to blame for your own misfortune/weight/empty wallet/dysfunctional relationships! That's not you, is it? When you live *at cause*, on the other hand, you give yourself choices.

Think of shows like *The X Factor, Britain's Got Talent* and *American Idol*. The contestants are living at cause – taking responsibility for trying to hit the big time. If they just sat at home waiting for their talents to be recognized, what would be their chances of getting a record deal? Or think of Nelson Mandela – he made the decision that 27 years of confinement would never take away his dignity. What would have happened if he'd decided to play the victim instead?

A Word about Identity

The choices we make are actually all about our identity – how we see ourselves, what we believe about ourselves, how we perceive our place in the world. When a decision fits our identity, we immediately know what to do, and we do it without question. Sportspeople, for example, have their nutrition and exercise regimes to follow, and it's not hard for them because it's part of their identity, but imagine how hard these same regimes would be for an office worker. Similarly, ballet dancers, athletes and jockeys know what nutritional programme to follow and it's not a struggle of willpower for them, it simply fits their identity. Professional musicians don't complain about the hours and hours of practice, getting that piece of music just right – again, it simply fits their identity.

Actors know that part of their identity is to look a particular way for a particular role, so they even lose or gain weight as required (like Renée Zellweger for *Bridget Jones' Diary*), without the struggle of ordinary mortals who aren't paid a few million dollars per movie. That's because to fulfil their identity as great actors, they will do whatever it takes. (Interestingly, identity is far more powerful than money: if a film bombs, do the millions earned make up for it?)

Natalie Portman recently trained five hours a day for months, swam several miles a day and followed a strict vegan diet in order to be able to dance like a professional ballet dancer in the acclaimed movie *The Black Swan*. She even misaligned a rib in the process! Did she complain? I doubt it! She was identifying with the character as closely as possible. Was she totally convincing in that movie? Yes. And the critics agree.

People who overeat often have a 'fat' identity. They want food to nurture them, but don't want to take the responsibility for nurturing themselves. It's almost a childlike state. Mum may not be there giving them the apple pie anymore, but the identity's still there when they eat for comfort. It's an identity that's at effect instead of at cause.

In this state, it's easier to blame the food or something else in life than to wake up and start taking responsibility for your actions. But when you shift your identity to being at cause, there are no excuses. You start taking responsibility for loving and respecting yourself through your actions and beliefs, no matter what is happening around you.

I had a client who told me:

> 'I worked in the fashion media and even at size 12 [US size 6], I thought I was fat. My identity was fat, because everyone else was so skinny. Because I thought I was fat, day after day I behaved like a fat person. Then I became fat. I made myself into the fat person I had in my mind. That's why I am now 22 stone [308 pounds]. The irony is I now realize that I originally wasn't fat at all! I'd do anything to get back to that old weight...'

Thing is, the client believed she was fat even *before* she started to work in the fashion industry. It's possible that her choice of career simply served to confirm that identity. That's why *identity* is so important and powerful. You really can create yourself in your own image, for good or ill.

As Dr Isaac Jones explained in the foreword of this book, he calls those who make a conscious choice to create an identity of health in body and mind 'lifestylers'. Lifestylers make a conscious choice to align their food and exercise and lifestyle choices around the identity of optimum health. I'd like to wager they wouldn't find turning down a huge slice of sweetened caramelized apple pie with sugared pastry crust and lashings of thick vanilla custard difficult – eating this type of food on a regular basis simply doesn't fit with their *identity*! It's not that they don't have comfort food, by the way – it's just not about sugar! Instead it's healthy, light and tasty food that gives them the sense of comfort that they are following their goals to be slim and fit and in optimum health. My personal comfort food is a big glass of water. It reassures me I'm hydrated and therefore setting myself up for optimum performance mentally and physically!

So, start questioning your identity to see if it is helping or hindering your health, fitness and weight-loss goals. Identity is powerful. As you go through this book, from time to time step back and ask yourself, 'What is my identity? How can I transform it for the best?'

We all have the potential to transform our identity and achieve more in life. Do you know that between two and four million bits of data stream into our unconscious mind *per second*? Or that we only consciously process around 134 bits per second – a really tiny fraction? [3] So we *all* have great untapped potential.

What makes the difference is how we use this brainpower. That's why the Keys in this book open a new way of thinking. You'll realize most of it is simply common sense; it's just thinking in ways you haven't thought before.

Shall I share a secret with you, one that has been proven time and time again in my years of business and training? The more flexibility you have, the more control you have, *the more solutions you will find and the greater your chance of success will be.*[4] *You* are the real key to unlocking your own success, and that's got to be your starting-point.

So … are you ready?

1

Before You Start

I once dated someone who constantly criticized my appearance. For five long years I felt shorter, fatter, uglier, less glamorous and less attractive than everyone else. I felt awful! My frantic search for the 'right' haircut, the 'right' clothes and the 'right' weight went on and on. My aim in life was to make my boyfriend happy, but I was deeply unhappy myself. When I hit rock-bottom, I finally booted him out. Just taking that *action* was a boost in self-esteem!

I realize now it wasn't his fault, because *hurt people hurt people.*[1] But a word of warning: if you want to lose weight for someone else, it won't work. You'll be resentful and that will sabotage the process. So ask yourself who you are doing this for. Everything's easier when you do it *for yourself* because know you deserve it! And when you love yourself, everything becomes easy. That's the most important lesson I have *ever* learned, and the reason I wrote this book.

However, it's OK to do something for yourself *as well as* 'because of' someone else. Note the difference: you're not doing it *for* someone else but *because of* someone else. That's a mother who'd like to lose weight *because of* her kids – she wants to be able to run around more with them. That's a husband who wants to stop drinking too much *because of* his family's concern about his liver problem. Both these people are motivated to make a change because they've realized how their behaviour is affecting those they care for. They're taking action from a 'place' of positivity, concern and unconditional love for self and others. Unlike me – I was trying to lose weight just to make my insecure boyfriend love me more!

The 3Cs and 2Rs

So, now you're sure you're doing this for yourself, what is it you're actually doing? And is it working? If not, you need to change to a new strategy. And you need to try out as many new strategies as possible until you find the one that works fantastically for you.

Let's suppose that the strategies you've used in the past to lose weight haven't worked. If you're reading this book, it's a fair assumption, isn't it? So what you need is a change in outlook and a change in behaviour.

Change +Action = Progress

Write that down and remember it!
And while you're taking action, you also need:

The **3 Cs:**

> *commitment*
>
> *congruency*
>
> *consistency*

Write those down as well!
Because to achieve success you have to:
- Start with *commitment.*
- Make sure you are supporting your cause by being *congruent*
  – that is, 'in agreement or harmony'.[2]
- Take action *consistently.*

There's another 'C' that's very important, too, as you take your first step towards successful weight loss: being *content* with the task ahead.

This means being kind to yourself by taking action *every day* to make yourself a happier and more fulfilled person. It also means having a weight-loss goal that includes:

The 2Rs:

> *realistic*
>
> *reasonable*

Write those down too.

Realistic means not aiming to become Michelle Pfeiffer if you weren't born with her genes! Aim instead to become a healthier, slimmer and more confident version of yourself.

Reasonable means being patient. You can't change everything at once. Take baby steps. Remember that new habits or behaviour need time.

Reasonable also means not beating yourself up if you slip up, but remembering to *keep calm and carry on*!

So, a successful strategy for weight loss involves:

1. *Accepting* that you need to lose weight.
2. *Committing* to losing weight. Commitment is a powerful boost of energy to help you on your way!
3. Having a *realistic* and *reasonable* weight-loss goal, both on a daily basis and in the long term. (It's important that the process is sustainable.)
4. *Enjoying* the ride: enjoying what you have achieved as well as looking forward to what you're going to achieve!

The Power of Seven Questions

The number seven is very powerful, so here are seven questions to help you understand where you're starting from and how you can make immediate progress. Take pen and paper and answer them straight away. These are life-changing questions, so please answer them with *commitment*.

Seven Questions to Target your Needs

1. 'Why do I want to lose weight?'
2. 'What need(s) will I be fulfilling by losing weight?'
3. 'What need(s) have I been fulfilling by *not* losing weight/ by eating too much?'
4. 'How can I fulfil those needs in a way that will serve me positively?'
5. 'Why do I eat certain foods?'

6. *'What* needs do I fulfil by eating these foods?'
7. *'How* can I fulfil those needs in a way that will serve me positively?'

If you want even more clarity, here's a more detailed set of questions to help you to get to the root of your actions. You can use them for weight loss or any other goal:

Seven Questions to Target your Actions

1. *'What* am I doing to help myself achieve my goal?'
2. *'What* am I *not* doing to help myself to achieve my goal?'
3. *'How* do I feel about what I'm *not* doing now?'
4. *'What* can I do instead to help myself achieve my goal?' (*Note:* Not 'What *could* I do?' The language is important.)
5. *'What* will I start doing right *now* to help myself achieve my goal?'
6. *'Where* will this lead and *how* do I feel about it?'
7. *'How* can I personalize the process so that it can be as fun and as easy as possible?'

To get the most out of using the Keys we're going to be looking at next, here are seven questions to enable you to understand and take control of your behaviour. Don't worry if this looks a lot of questions, by the way – you can always concentrate on just one set per week.

Seven Questions to Take Control

1. *'Why* do I indulge in actions I wish to change/behaviour that does not serve me?'
2. *'Why* need(s) am I fulfilling by doing this?'
3. *'What* can I choose to do instead?'
4. *'How* can I fulfil my need(s) in a healthier way that will serve me?'
5. *'How* can I change my strategy or behaviour to go about things in a different way?'
6. *'Can* I look at my behaviour from a different angle?'
7. *'Who* will I need to become to put these healthy strategies into practice?'

And seven questions to provide you with new and positive strategies:

Seven Questions to Provide Strategies for Success

1. '*What* are my seven new strategies for getting where I want to be?'
2. '*What* are my seven targeted *actions* to take in the next seven days?'
3. '*How* can I personalize my eating plan to best serve me? Can I do without something or do I have to work with it in a different way or quantity so that it nurtures me?'
4. '*How* can I modify or adjust as I go along to ensure I'm meeting my needs as well as my aims?'
5. '*How* can I *Track, Test and Treat* these achievements –*Track progress, Test results and Treat myself* for achieving milestones?'
6. '*How much* do I want this?' (Ask yourself daily.)
7. '*What* will I be missing out on if I don't achieve what I'm aiming for?' (Ask yourself daily.)

And finally, take a while to think about what motivates you:

Seven Labels to Understand What Motivates You

Jot down the seven labels below on a piece of paper and write down *everything* you associate with them:

1. 'Identity' and/or 'Security'
2. 'Ease'
3. 'Pleasure' and/or 'Comfort'
4. 'Time'
5. 'Knowledge' and/or 'Responsibility'
6. 'Commitment'
7. 'Vision' (your goals)

Then take a second piece of paper. Write down what these words would mean to you if you applied them to your weight-loss goal (you can do this with any goal in your life).

Your answers will give you insight into your individual belief system (the way *you* think). Study them carefully: understanding your motives is key to your success. You will begin to understand the strategies that you use unthinkingly to control your behaviour. And once you understand your thoughts and motivations in this way, you can devise new and positive strategies!

The 28 Keys that follow will help you to do this and open the door not only to weight-loss success, but to much more…

So, as you prepare to turn those Keys, let me wish you *good luck*! Do you know that 'luck' stands for 'Labouring Under Correct Knowledge'?

But first, a very important note…

Important: Seek Help If You Need It

If you suspect you have an eating disorder, do seek help, because the diseases anorexia and bulimia nervosa aren't success, they're failure. Organ failure, eventually…

My best friend at school became anorexic after her boyfriend dumped her. Perhaps she wanted to become more attractive? Who knows, but she ended up losing her looks, health and education. She nearly died at sweet 16. Was it worth it? I can picture her now – those sad, empty eyes. It's because of her that I set out on a quest to teach myself nutrition and behavioural psychology, even when I was still working in banks. It's because of her that I wrote this book.

Deep down, beyond the denial and lies, anorexics and bulimics always know the truth of their condition. They depend on taking control of their lives by controlling their eating. But it's an illusion!

Look at the side-effects of eating disorders: an abnormally slow heart rate (bradycardia); unusually low blood pressure (hypotension); disturbances in the heart rhythm (arrhythmia); reduction in the work capacity of the heart; heart muscle starvation and cardiomyopathy (inability of the heart muscle to pump blood, leading to fatality); gastrointestinal complications, including constipation, abdominal pain, dehydration and haemorrhoids; changes to enzyme levels and possible liver damage; disruption in thyroid function; hormonal changes; unbalanced thyroid and growth hormones; high cholesterol; restricted blood flow; osteopenia (loss of bone minerals); osteoporosis (loss of bone mass); increased risk of bone fracture; metabolic alkalosis (imbalance in the acid/base balance in the body); hypokalaemia (low potassium level) and other electrolyte imbalance (which can have life-threatening consequences); anaemia; pneumonia and respiratory disease; ruptured oesophagus or stomach lining; stomach ulcers; acid reflux; sleep apnoea (stopping breathing while asleep); suppressed immunity; dry, flaky skin with perhaps a yellow tinge; fine, downy hair on the face, back, arms and legs; possible loss of hair on the head; brittle nails; erosion of dental enamel leading to tooth loss; convulsions; coma; and, eventually, organ failure leading to *death*.

Psychological effects include: stress; depression; social withdrawal and difficulties with inter-personal interaction; irritability; sleep disruption and fatigue; decreased concentration span; affective (mood) disorders; anxiety disorders; personality disorders and other addictions or compulsions. Some individuals even display symptoms that meet the diagnostic criteria for a major depressive disorder.[3]

If you think these side-effects 'happen to someone else', how about these:

- excessive body and facial hair
- halitosis (bad breath)
- amenorrhoea (lack of menstrual cycle leading to potential infertility)
- muscle wastage

Think these will make you more attractive? *Think again*!

The serious medical side-effects of anorexia and bulimia nervosa are not to be underestimated. Note that they include death.

Eating disorders are no different from substance abuse and are just as addictive. If you think you have an eating disorder, do seek professional help before it is too late. You can trust medical professionals to treat you with courtesy and confidentiality. Eating disorders are beyond my professional scope and require, I repeat, proper medical intervention from a qualified healthcare professional in the field of eating disorders.

In the United Kingdom, try **www.anorexiabulimiacare.org.uk or sufferers' helpline: 01934 710679 and parents' helpline: 01934 710645.**

Also, please note that if you are suffering from depression or any form of mental health issue or have a diagnosed or suspected illness or dependency on drugs, narcotics, medication, alcohol or tobacco products or are prone to self-harming episodes, then losing weight will *not* suddenly resolve any self-esteem issues you may be facing.

If you are suffering from any of the above, you are strongly advised to seek the advice of a medical doctor or appropriate health professional, as the advice in this book is not designed to replace proper professional medical advice or counselling and is not intended to medically treat any condition which is best dealt with by the relevant healthcare professional.

This warning is important and necessary, of course, but hopefully not relevant for the vast majority of you, who are looking forward eagerly with healthy optimism to a positive change of mindset and behaviour, and to increased health and vitality in both mind and body! So, let's turn the key in the door which leads to slimming success and read on…

2

28 Keys to Thinking Differently

Here are 28 Keys to open the door to an improved body shape and greater confidence!

This is how to use them:

1. Read one Key at a time and *apply it*. If you ever find the fit less than perfect, move on and come back to it when you're ready. Take one step at a time: 'a journey of a thousand miles starts with a single step'.[1] Each step will take you closer to your goal, and you'll realize how simple it is to *take control* as your energy levels and your morale increase right from the word *go!*

2. This is not *just* about losing weight: this is a lifetime process of self-maximization! You want to make the most of yourself, don't you, and that means body, soul, mind and spirit! So, while applying the Keys to your life, think of how you can use your energy positively to do *other* interesting or profitable things too. Before you know it, you'll be losing weight as a sideline of expanding your heart and mind and ... possibly ... wallet. Do you know that it's when you first serve yourself and then start to serve others that you really attract wealth into your life?

3. Individualize the Keys. Use them in the context of your own life. Recall what you personally have done in the past and concentrate on the changes you personally are going to make *from now on!*

4. Visualize, visualize, *visualize!* Visualization is creating a picture or movie in your mind. Visualizing performing an action daily enables you to do it naturally and easily when you're ready. This works because your unconscious mind doesn't differentiate between what's real and what's vividly imagined. Top sportspeople and performers use this technique all the time. You think of an actual situation in as much vivid detail as possible, picturing yourself there, achieving your goal. For weight loss, you can imagine yourself at your favourite restaurant table, choosing nutritious food and savouring each mouthful slowly, or making healthy food and exercise choices. The more you make the pictures colourful, loud, vivid and *real*, engaging all your senses, the more effective this technique is. It's not a trick, believe me: it's a powerful tool for positive change. Your unconscious mind responds to the realistic pictures and movies you create on its screen, believes they are real and acts accordingly!

5. Practise, practise, practise! Musicians and sportspeople have to practise new techniques and the rest of us are no different! Practise each Key day after day until it becomes easy and effortless. Practise your visualizations – your little movies of living, eating and feeling your ideal shape, health and energy level – at least three to four times a day. Practice makes perfect!

6. You can go through the Keys one by one or just choose at random, but do be serious about each one. These are tools to empower you to make serious changes. *Be ambitious* – that is, *know* that you're going to take action to achieve results, *choose* to take action to achieve results and then, quite simply, *do it!*

Your journey starts here, so here we go, and good luck, you have the power to create a brand new body, with confidence and self-confidence to boot! And who knows what more besides? It's all up to you. What a wonderful journey you're going to have, creating yourself in your brand new image, your new identity…

Key Number One

Build Up Good Habits, Remove Bad Ones

How long do you think it takes to form a habit? And what *is* a habit anyway?

My *Concise Oxford English Dictionary*'s definition is: 'a settled or regular tendency or practice'. And the *Oxford English Dictionary* also has an old-fashioned definition: 'a person's *health* or *constitution…*' (my italics).

It has been found that it's the 'regular' part of a habit that's important. Behaviour needs to be repeated to become 'settled' or automatic – like a toddler learning to sit on the potty!

Now for the science behind it. In his book *Psycho-cybernetics*, Dr Maxwell Maltz explained that it took 21 days for amputees to stop feeling 'phantom' sensations in the place where an amputated limb used to be. From this starting-point he deduced that it took 21 days to create a new pattern of thinking.[2] Since a habit is quite simply *a new pattern of thinking*, you can therefore create a new one in 21 days!

We all know that the longer you do something, the more it becomes automatic – like driving or even learning to walk. But sometimes we're not quite so aware of how we're creating habits day after day. We pride ourselves on going to the gym regularly: that's a good habit! But what about reaching for that snack when our favourite TV show's on? What type of habit is that?

If you love a snack – say, crisps – what do you love exactly: the texture, the taste, the crunch? You might associate the taste with good times and pleasure and relaxation. But have you ever noticed that the crunch is kind of oily? That oily crunch is actually what makes that crisp so unhealthy! Every bite releases fatty calories into your mouth. Then those calories travel to your hips and sit there, and won't budge easily! They hold you hostage to hours at the gym and too-tight jeans!

A client of mine thought about this and every time she sat down to watch TV she imagined the crispy calories were evil crispy little gremlins conspiring to fatten her up! Soon she was no longer reaching for the crisps and was drinking sparkling water instead!

All she'd done was change her pattern of thinking. Instead of thinking about how nice those snacks were, she'd started imagining all the nasty consequences. When she'd thought about those consequences for long enough, day after day, she'd created a new habit: *not* eating crisps in front of the TV!

So, how are habits formed? Let's go a bit into the background of how we learn. The brain creates connections (synapses or neural pathways) between brain cells (neurons), which are like a roadmap for learning information or behaviour. You can imagine them as short-cuts. Without going into detail, the most accepted theory on the working of the brain today is called 'Hebbian Learning', which summarizes that 'Neurons that fire together wire together.'[3] Quite a jingle, isn't it?

All this sounds quite technical and your neurons are probably overloaded already! But it's actually just like learning the route to a particular destination: the *neurons* are your landmarks and the *synapses* are the roads which link them. When you're in an unfamiliar part of town, you concentrate on watching out for the landmarks on the way. But if you drive past them on a regular basis then you know the way 'instinctively'. But it's not instinct at all – it's learned behaviour. It's your brain coding the route, running a little mini program every time you have to get from that particular A to that particular B. The more your brain runs the same pattern of connections, the more you're making it automatic and permanent. This is how you learn.

On the other hand, to *break* an established habit, you have to make the route *less effective*. You can do this by reprogramming the pattern of behaviour that created the habit in the first place – basically, by doing something different. This has the effect of weakening the synapse (the established link).

Furthermore, when you change established behaviour, you need to put new behaviour in its place – bright yellow diversion signs to take you in a new direction! The more you substitute the new behaviour, the weaker the old route becomes. But, unlike the yellow signs, you can't take the new behaviour away, or the old behaviour will return – which is why just one drink or cigarette can be disastrous for those training their brains to quit craving alcohol or nicotine.

My husband is always telling me to 'break the pattern' when I nag at him to pick up his smelly socks. Trouble is, he never suggests substitute behaviour for the nagging. So do you think I quit nagging and break the pattern?!

Another way to break the link is to make the outcome undesirable. This is like training dogs not to poop on the floor by tapping them on the nose with a rolled-up newspaper every time they do it. But motivation is generally more effective than punishment. Punishment causes resentment and dissatisfaction – which is why diets don't work!

Which of these two options sounds nicer to you:

> 'If you eat that doughnut, you'll be fat, miserable and guilty.'
> 'If you refuse that doughnut, you'll feel slim, healthy and empowered!'

And which do you think gets better results?

So, the best way to harness the power of the mind is to repeat positive actions and thoughts daily. Now I'm not talking about repeating affirmations in front of the mirror, though this can help some people, I'm talking about making a change to your thinking patterns and practising those changes every day.

Remember: *change + action = progress*!

It's *consistency* that's important here. We all know that if you change your eating habits for the duration of a diet but then revert, the weight lost will creep back on. Why? Like the thermostat controlling temperature in your house, the 'ponderostat' [4] in your body carries the in-built 'memory' of your optimum (read 'famine-proof' and 'fattest') body weight, to which you'll return to time and time again unless you reset its calibration over a longer term. This is why 'quick fixes' and 'crash diets' don't work! You may be forcing your body to burn fat in famine mode, but you're doing nothing to re-route the behavioural patterns that created the fat in the first place!

That's why when you're changing established neurological patterns, you need to commit to being consistent, trusting that the new route to a better habit is being carved out day after day after day. Until eventually the new thoughts and actions become so easy they appear effortless.

So, how are we going to put all this theory into practice?

You're going to make one positive change, like quitting snacking in front of the TV and drinking sparkling water instead (but please do personalize it), for a calendar month – 28, 30 or 31 days. Mark up your calendar and promise yourself that you'll make the change for the duration – no more, no less.

This is not about forcing yourself: it's a holiday, an experience of something different, an opportunity to go a new route! It's your chance to realize how easy it is to re-route a pattern of behaviour. And once you've made that first decision, it'll become easier ... and easier ... and easier...

Then, on the first day of the following month, ask yourself, how you feel. If you feel oh, so much better, then you can easily keep on going, can't you? You see, after your initial commitment, it can feel effortless!

What you've done in this exercise is wired yourself to behave in a way which will serve you better.

Now take pen and paper and write this down:

> *The decisions I make and the actions I take determine my "wiring".'*

Consider this quote from the Dutch Renaissance humanist and theologian Desiderius Erasmus: 'A nail is driven out by another nail; habit is overcome by habit.'[5]

Key Points to Remember
- It takes 21 days for the brain to learn a new habit.
- Make a positive change consistently every day and you will be re-routing your thought patterns and your behaviour.
- Once the new route is consolidated, it will become effortless.
- New habits are simply new wiring in the brain.
- The decisions you make and the actions you take determine your 'wiring'.
- 'A nail is driven out by another nail; habit is overcome by habit.'

Key Number Two

How to Manage Change

Do you *really* want to lose weight? Are you *truly* aiming to get fitter? You might think you are, but have you ever felt unsure or uncomfortable about what change might bring? If I told you you were going to get the body of a porn star, would you feel just a *little* uncomfortable? Most of the women I tested this on did. The men? I won't say! But many people don't like the association – and they won't aspire to something they don't feel comfortable with.

Many people even sabotage their weight-loss aspirations because they identify so much with being overweight that they can't see themselves as slim! It just seems too much of a leap in identity. Some are worried they'll be forced to put in daily sessions on the treadmill to maintain a new weight. Others are scared of their partner's reaction when they 'turn into someone else', or are secretly scared of 'out-slimming' their wife or husband!

Do you know what's so sad about this? It's missing the point. You don't need to turn into Arnold Schwarzenegger or Pamela Anderson just because you lose some weight – honestly! How about simply turning into a healthier, fitter, slimmer version of *your very own self*?

It can only ever be *good* to improve your health and your looks and your fitness. Don't ever let anyone tell you otherwise. Be pleased to make the most of yourself. No one will love you less for it – and if they do, they're just jealous, that's the bottom line.

Yes, sadly there are always losers intent on sabotaging other people's success. It's an unfortunate fact of life that many people are scared of success and instead of seeking it themselves they'll try to sabotage other people's so they don't end up feeling inferior. So, be aware that those closest to you may suffer jealousy, feelings of competition and a sense of threat if you decide to make a change. Even friends and family may, out of a misdirected sense of 'protection', try to sabotage your plans, making comments like:

> 'Nonsense, you are fine the way you are. We all have a few extra pounds.'

> 'It wouldn't suit you to be skinny.'

> 'Why bother with the hassle? Just enjoy these chips.'

> 'Don't believe all this stuff you read in books.'

> 'None of the family's slim – you're just heavy-boned like the rest of us.'

> 'Where do you want to lose weight – on your eyelashes?!'

> 'Oh, so you want to ruin our meals together by not eating!'

Ignore it! Be polite but firm and go your own way. Do your own thing. Leave the loser mentality behind. Ask the naysayers or the saboteurs if there is anything wrong in improving yourself. Get them to acknowledge that change for the better *is* better! How can they refuse that logic? Those who care for you will surely come round to it and be happy for you once you've succeeded. If not, they are just not *yet* ready to acknowledge and support your growth, so distance yourself from them, while being respectful of their right to an opinion, and always leave them with the chance to come round in the future. Remember it's likely to be all about *them* rather than about *you*, so don't take it personally!

Of course it's natural to be scared of change, to feel fear around a new project, to wonder if you're up to accepting a positive transformation. We're all human. We're programmed for survival, and a fear of change is part of that – it's designed to protect us in a risky environment. The problem is that coupled with the desire for comfort and familiarity, it can sabotage the best of intentions!

My favourite book title is Susan Jeffers' *Feel the Fear and Do It Anyway*. Because *beyond* the fear of change, of failure, of the unknown, lies the *promised land of opportunity and improvement!* And it's worth any effort to get there.

In any case, fear of the unknown is only in the mind.

Repeat after me:

'Fear of the unknown is only in the mind. All it is is fear of fear!'

Now take pen and paper and write it down.

It's important to know that when you're scared of the unknown, what you're really scared of is just *fear itself*, which exists ... that's right ... you know ... *only* in your own mind...

Can you think of a time when you were worried that something would be really tough? And then, once you got started, it was pretty easy after all?

In an article for the *Sunday Telegraph*'s women's supplement 'Stella', journalist Sarra Manning considered whether losing weight really was 'the magic formula to happiness'. It was a question she could answer from personal experience, as she had weighed more than 25 stone (350 pounds) six years earlier and had since lost more than 150lb. She wrote:

> 'I had a nagging suspicion that all my doubt and uncertainty
> weren't going to miraculously disappear just because I
> could get into a size 10 [US size 2] Marc Jacobs dress. ...If
> I wasn't fat anymore, then I had nothing to hide behind. If
> being a size 14 wasn't the solution then *I* was the problem....
> [But] if I'd never been fat, then I'd never have gained the
> power and knowledge that come with transformation.'[6]

Remember the 2 Rs? It's precisely because Sarra's outlook was so *realistic* and *reasonable* that she lost so much weight. She didn't expect miracles overnight. She accepted herself, with all her faults, right from the start. She felt the fear and did it anyway. And achieved massive results and success! When you *do* leap off your backside and embrace change, all sorts of good things start to happen. What would you like to happen to you? Would you like to enjoy a different view? Meet new people? Learn new things? Discover the world?

First you have to make a change. Then, once you get into the flow, things will get easier. Whatever worries you had will quite simply drop away!

No journey should be scary, because there are no right or wrong roads to get to your destination. As long as you keep moving in the right direction, you can always adjust your route. In fact, there are usually multiple ways to get there. Remember, *the more solutions to a problem, the more chances of success!*

If I'd been scared of change, you wouldn't be reading this book. When I first had the idea, years and years ago, I had no qualifications to write it, I had no experience, no publisher and no real idea how to go about it. I just had a helluva lot of passion and ambition. So I put pen to paper, bum to seat, and hoped for the best! It flowed: I adjusted, learned, studied, got qualifications, became an expert, networked, got contacts, a publisher, adjusted and revised and revised again … and here you are!

It's the ability to be flexible when aiming for a goal that distinguishes not only world-class footballers like David ('Bend it') Beckham, but anyone who's successful. Mega-bestselling author Jeffrey Archer goes through on average 17 drafts for every book that he writes [7] – and that's a lot of adjustment (believe me, I know)! But the principle is the same for any project – you have to start and then adjust along the way.

One thing that many people are scared of is that making a change will mean they have to be someone or something they are not. But losing a spot of weight doesn't mean you suddenly have to become glamorous if instead you feel more casual, or outspoken if you feel shy! You don't suddenly have to turn into a sex god or goddess if inside you feel more like a nun or priest (don't laugh, some of us actually do sometimes!) You can still be yourself. And what's so wonderful is that you'll be a *healthier and more comfortable version of yourself.*

Change is liberating. When you make a change to improve yourself, you lose what I call 'worry weight'. You don't need to worry that you need to improve – you *are* improving. Now isn't that a *weight off your shoulders?* Doesn't it improve your confidence and your mood? And give you more energy? And make you more fun to be around? There's simply no downside to positive change!

So instead of worrying that a change might be painful or scary, ask yourself, 'Will this change free up worry weight? And what can I use that energy for instead?'

Here are some case studies to give you a few ideas:

Prianka

Prianka, 35, who works in IT, went from a size 22 (US 16) to a size 12 (US 6), using a carefully tailored vegetarian diet and the Keys in this book. At the beginning, she could barely walk to the shops without feeling out of breath. Now she has the confidence to go to the gym and go swimming in stretchy outfits she'd never dreamed of wearing before!

Prianka's friends and associates are full of compliments about her newfound energy and motivation: she's an inspiration to everyone to get fitter. All her self-consciousness is gone – with everybody so full of praise for her transformation, she's glowing with confidence!

Now Prianka's no longer hiding behind an overweight 'front', she's motivated to make the very most of herself. She's on a roll, feeling that she really does *deserve* it. And there's nothing more rewarding than feeling that you deserve something!

Nathalie

Nathalie, 28, who works in a bank, has this story to tell:

> 'I used to date a guy who was really jealous – always telling me what to wear and what not to wear. And I work in a pretty conservative environment – it's all dark suits and pinstripes! So I started to dress plainly, which really isn't me at all. I guess on some level I was scared of being judged.

> Then I started to put on weight. I didn't think much of it. But it got to the point where it was really affecting my self-confidence – what was left of it.

> Working through the reasons with my Neurostrategist, I discovered it was all because of *fear*. I was scared to upset my boyfriend. I was scared my boss wouldn't approve of me. I was scared of rocking the boat. I was scared of being myself! Putting on weight meant I didn't have the option of dressing sassy! It was kind of forcing me into a new, dull, identity so I didn't have to be scared anymore! Perverse, what your mind can do.

> Being scared of success is more common than you'd think. I come across it all the time at work. Many of the guys are very successful, earning big bucks, flashing the cash. But then on some level they self-sabotage: drinking too much, eating too much, overspending, even drugs sometimes – it's almost as

though they're trying to bring themselves back down to earth.

I decided to hell with it. If I couldn't be
myself, what was the point?

So I ditched the dead-end boyfriend and started wearing
brighter colours. I quit being scared of being a little bit
different. No one cared, of course, because as my confidence
went up, my performance at work did too. And I got a really
great pay rise! Now I've got a reason to walk in grinning
every day – and I've even been in talks with someone to
help me invest in a new business idea: I'm thinking about
designing work wear with a difference – brighter colours
and cheeky little details for female execs who don't want
to be conservative! I've always wanted to be my own boss
and now it looks as though it might really happen!'

Here's a simple little Neurostrategy technique – that's a strategy for
advanced behavioural optimization and change – that I've modified for
you. It will enable you to set a single goal into your mind and remove any
fear attached to it. It will help you to achieve it easily and effortlessly, so
that change becomes *comfortable* for you!

I'll go through the steps. Read through them and follow them carefully:

1. Ask yourself: 'What is the *last thing* that has to happen so I
   really know I'm here [at my ideal weight/fitness level]?' When
   you ask yourself this question, you are accessing your own
   'evidence criteria' - your own 'proof' that you've reached
   your goal. Visualize whatever it is that best represents
   your proof. For example, I imagine myself standing in my
   bedroom, doing up my tightest, smallest, skinniest jeans
   comfortably without a struggle! *Now fix your picture of your
   unique 'proof' in your mind.*

2. Now, access this picture (we call it an 'internal representation')
   each and every day without fail. Make it as *big*, as *bright*,
   as *vivid* and as *real* as you possibly can! (Remember the
   unconscious mind can't tell the difference between what
   is real and what is vividly imagined.) *See the colours, hear
   the sounds, feel the textures, smell the aromas, feel the
   feelings...* (Spring air or summer sunshine, compliments of
   a shop assistant, strength and lightness and freedom, the

little voice inside saying, 'Yeah, baby, you look great!' – those are mine. What are yours?)

3. Now, just to be sure, adjust the colours to the *brightest*, the sounds to the *loudest*, all the senses to the *most vivid*, the feelings to the *most positive* and *most real* – go right up as far as you can go. Crank up the dials up to the max, baby!

4. When you've accessed the picture and made it as *vivid* and *real* as possible, *step out of it so that you are looking at it (and yourself in it), from the outside in.*

5. When you are looking at the picture from the outside in, take it in your hands and imagine floating up above yourself, above where you are sitting or standing, above the current moment, like a bird into the air.

6. Energize the picture with four deep breaths, breathing in through your nose and out through your mouth, and blow all your energy into your picture: *Haaaa...*

7. Now, energized, float out above yourself into your future – wherever you picture your future to be located in your mind is great. When you are there, let go of the picture and let it float right down into your future, like a leaf floating down to the earth, full of the life energy you've filled it with.

8. Notice the events between that point in the future and the point where you are now shift to support your goal. You needn't see the details, just know that all the actions and circumstances and situations between then and now are shifting to support you in your mission.

9. Your mission is complete, so float back to the present moment. Your goal is set in your future and your unconscious mind has received all the instructions you need to assist you in attaining it!

10. You must visualize your 'proof' three or four times a day. *The picture is the instruction you are giving to your unconscious mind.* You're telling yourself what you want to become - and your mind is helping you along the way! Say to yourself: 'Knowing how great I feel about achieving my goal, how much am I going to *enjoy the ride* as I *notice my progress* and *circumstances shifting to support my goal* along the way and carry me along to success?!'

Key Points to Remember
- *Don't ever* be afraid of making a change for the better!
- If friends, family or acquaintances try to sabotage your plans for self-improvement, be polite but firm and go your own way. Leave the loser mentality behind.
- Distance yourself from people who do not support your goals, while being respectful of their right to an opinion. Remember it's more likely to be about *them* than about *you.*
- Do what you want to do for yourself, and for yourself only. If you are making a change for anyone else, it may not end up being sustainable in the longer term.
- Once you get into the flow, things will get easier. Whatever worries you had will quite simply drop away!

Key Number Three

When Pain is Gain

When I was giving birth to my daughter I had to learn very quickly to accept the pain and work with it. It was a great lesson for life, but the steepest learning curve I've ever come across! There was no time for pain-relief medication, so I had no choice. But as soon as I acknowledged that pain was going to be part of the process and welcomed it as an essential part of producing my much-wished-for baby girl, something truly magical happened: it no longer had any power over me! I was listening to my body and understanding what was going to happen and what the discomfort was all about, and it was as if I'd moved onto a different plane of existence where I could feel the pain to a certain extent yet I wasn't a slave to it. I had a degree of objectivity and freedom from suffering. This feeling of control was far more powerful than all the pain relief I'd been given 20 months before, at the birth of my son!

The difference was that in allowing myself to truly feel during my daughter's birth, I gained understanding, objectivity and control. At my son's birth, on the other hand, I was totally at effect of everything. I was drugged up to the nines with pain-relief medication, yet you'll have figured out by now which birth was the more traumatic!

The strength I've taken from this experience has served me ever since. To be able to listen to your mind and body fully and calmly, no matter how much emotion or discomfort tries to distract you, gives you immense power. You are both fully in the moment but objective at the same time. It's a huge resource to have against pain and fear and discomfort. You don't even need to give birth to develop it! Sportspeople and ballet dancers work through pain all the time when they train and perform. Some even say that pain gives them an edge.

Now I'm not suggesting you start to push yourself physically to the limit and become a martyr – quite the opposite! This Key is all about being quiet and calm. It's about developing the ability to pause and allow yourself quite simply to *feel*. It's about listening to your feelings, both physical and emotional, *without* fighting them. It's about looking beyond pain and understanding it so that it loses its power over you.

Our modern world is all about increasing comfort and reducing discomfort. Yet many more traditional societies do not attempt to anaesthetize emotional pain. In fact, with no therapists to turn to, difficult emotions are more readily expressed! This can lead to them being released and resolved. There's a word for the healing nature of letting out emotion: 'cathartic'. Uncomfortable feelings are, after all, there for a reason: the unconscious mind is trying to communicate something important! So, by taking notice of your uncomfortable feelings, you learn more about yourself. And you realize that strength lies in understanding and accepting yourself – every facet of yourself. This realization is immensely powerful, because when you understand rather than struggle, you *take back control*. When you know the nature of the beast, you can tame it!

As we already know, familiarity gives us comfort and pleasure. It's the unknown that can be scary. When you break a habit or make a change, you have to let go of what you know. This can feel uncomfortable, painful even. It's like a ballet dancer learning a new move. That can be painful to start off with, while the muscles are unfamiliar with the position. But that's life. It's by working through pain that new skills are learned.

It's the same with our minds. New habits can be just as much of a stretch and just as 'painful', but it is mental muscle being tested instead of physical muscle!

So, when you are *itching* to reach for that snack even when you aren't physically hungry, or when you're feeling insecure and physically unattractive, or when you're feeling depleted of energy and unfit, the answer is to stop fighting the sensation and allow yourself to fully *feel* it.

By fully experiencing the emotion, you will find it becoming less powerful and having less of a hold on you. By not indulging in any activity designed to anaesthetize it, you are allowing it to take its natural course and serve its purpose. And by not fighting it, you are preserving precious energy. This energy can then be harnessed to find creative solutions!

Let's say you have a craving for chocolate. What happens if you ignore it and work through the feeling instead of reaching for a chocolate bar? By not giving into the craving, you've broken the chain reaction and given yourself a window of opportunity to see things objectively. Instead of munching away, you can be busy asking yourself *why* you had the craving in the first place and *what need* it was trying to fulfil.

Once you start to analyse your thoughts in this way, you will find the pain or discomfort passes. You regain power over your thoughts and your impulses. You overcome temptation by stepping back and letting it flutter away. You're back in control of your life and your actions! And doesn't that feel good?

I once had the fantastic experience of serving on a jury. It was a massive honour but also a daunting responsibility to have the fate of a fellow human being hanging on our judgement. The most important lesson we had to learn was that reason must always trump emotion. We had to learn to take a step back, review all the information objectively and make the soundest judgement possible according to the facts available.

We also had to learn to listen to our intuition. This is different from emotion. Emotion is easy to recognize – it's loud, bright and in your face. Intuition, often called the 'sixth sense', is like a tiny little voice hiding away beneath layers of thought. You have to give it space to make itself heard! Do give it space, always. It offers priceless information. It's your unconscious mind speaking to you!

My jury experience was a fantastic lesson for life. Would you feel comfortable being tried by a jury of 12 angry men or women following their emotions and not their logic? Yet every day inside our own minds many of us allow ourselves to be governed that way. We make judgements based on sudden emotion and impulsiveness. (*'Verdict? The accused is tired! She may eat that chocolate biscuit!'*) We forget to listen to what is really going on and don't try and understand it. Instead, it would be so much better for us to sit and quietly listen to the evidence before making up our own minds as to which course of action is best for us.

Sitting on that jury, there was often pain. You couldn't help thinking, 'That victim could be my father or my brother! My mother or my sister!' But we had to work through that pain and realize we weren't being objective. Because what if the person standing there accused of a crime were a relative too? Our job was to look behind the pain to find the truth.

So, if you're feeling sad, frustrated, insecure or angry, just sit and let the emotions flow and you'll find that the mind will quieten itself after the heady onslaught and you'll be better placed to put things into perspective. After the emotions have passed, you'll be able to look for the silver lining and remember that some *things* can't be changed, but your *perspective* can always be changed! When you are able to think rationally instead of emotionally, you have the space to review the situation, see things differently and recognize the opportunities opening up for you. When the mind is free of overwhelming emotion, you can finally listen to your intuition. And your unconscious mind, as we have learned, has immense resources at its disposal!

So, stop and listen – *really* listen – and then, instead of covering up your feelings with a cream cake or a doughnut, you'll know what to do.

Key Points to Remember
- Making a change or facing the unknown is a break from familiarity and comfort. But experience is power.
- By allowing ourselves to experience the discomfort of difficulty – either tough emotions or the challenge of breaking a habit – we are also allowing ourselves to gain experience, strength and objectivity.
- Just as pain in the body signals the need for healing, so pain in the mind signals a need for change.
- Allow the storm to pass and the mind to quieten and you'll gain inner strength.
- Be your own judge and jury. Use objectivity, not emotion, to understand yourself.
- When you truly listen to your feelings, you'll know what to do.

Key Number Four

Get What You Deserve

It's so easy to forget how lucky we really are. Across the world there are people who are suffering each and every day, including those living in the midst of war and conflict, those robbed of health and those faced with the illness or death of a loved one. In this context, what does being a little bit overweight matter?

My view is that we all deserve the very best of everything. Sadly, not everyone gets what they deserve. But for those of us who do have the opportunities and resources, not to take advantage of them is, quite frankly, a crying shame.

My mission is to teach the world to become healthier and fitter in mind, body and spirit! I believe that the happier and more balanced we are as individuals, the freer we can be as a society to look outside our own little world and serve others in a wider context.

The first step to making the most of the fantastic opportunities the world offers (and to help others to do so too) is to feel that we *deserve* them. Listen up – it's a very important concept! I speak from experience: it's only when I acknowledged that I deserved great things that they started to flow into my life!

So I'm going to ask you five really important questions…

Please take a few moments to grab pen and paper and answer these questions to the best of your ability. Really let the truth flow from within you. Write what you feel. Write what comes naturally.

1. Why do you want to lose weight and get fit? Do you feel you deserve to?
2. Do you believe you can do it easily?
3. If I say, 'Losing weight is a life or death situation for you,' what now? Can you do it easily now?
4. If you answered 'Yes' to question 3, what does that mean?
5. Are you in the privileged position of having all the resources to be healthy, slim and fit?

And now please answer these questions too:

1. What is the greatest way to honour those who do not have the opportunities and resources that you have?
2. Will you take advantage of the amazing opportunities and resources you have and not waste them?
3. What actions will you take now to honour the opportunities and gifts that you have been given as a privileged member of society who can afford the price of this book? Because for the price of this book I'm giving you the most cutting-edge techniques in the world today to assist you to make the most of yourself physically and, in doing so, to increase your self-confidence and boost your mood and general happiness!

But wait – there should be a warning attached to any promise that weight reduction will automatically guarantee happiness. I'm sure that we've all realized by now that being thin doesn't equal being happy, and being rich doesn't equal being happy either! Can you name a super-rich and super-thin celebrity (or two) who doesn't seem very happy?

Remember that happy people are slimmer, but slimmer people are not necessarily happier. *So make it your priority to be happy!*

I think it's fair to say that if you're rich, famous, good-looking, powerful and still self-sabotaging, then you've forgotten to be grateful for what you have. Gratitude for gifts and resources, simple little pleasures or greater ones, is the key to happiness. And the flip side of gratitude is accepting and acknowledging that you *deserve* what you've been given.

Take a moment each and every day to be *grateful* for what you have, recognizing that you *deserve* to have good things in your life, and the universe will listen to you and collaborate with you to give you even more. Believe it! It's not some hocus-pocus! I used to think it was, but then it worked for me and I witnessed it working for the many successful, fulfilled, wealthy and sometimes famous people I come into contact with on a daily basis.

If you're wondering what to be grateful for, well, if you've had the opportunity to purchase this book and you're sitting quietly reading it, then you probably live in a safe and abundant world. The fact that we enjoy these privileges gives us a duty of sorts to make the most of what we have. We need to take a few moments out of our busy schedule each day to reflect on how lucky we are. We are in such a fortunate position even compared to 25 years ago – even the richest man in the world then didn't have access to the information that we have at our fingertips on the internet every day!

Focusing on problems, on the other hand, only serves to bring more of the same. That's the way the universe works!

So, how about starting by appreciating what you have got and acknowledging what brings you wealth in all its senses, rather than focusing on what you *think* you haven't got? What's the point of whingeing about how you're not wealthy enough, for example? There are so many ways of being wealthy – starting with being healthy. Repeat after me: 'Wealth is health!'

Just recently, for instance, I read about a bride-to-be who died of heart failure after being on a restrictive diet of less than 600 calories a day to lose weight for her wedding. She never got to that wedding at all. That's a real lesson in perspective – a tragic one.

Some people look at the gap between themselves and celebrities and start to feel they could never measure up. Well, let me tell you something! Having met some of them, I really can say that they're just as human as the rest of us. Ali Campbell, celebrity life coach and a mentor to me, really hit the nail on the head when he told me, over a cup of coffee, 'Most celebrities are just ordinary people, but they're doing extraordinary jobs!' Remember that though they might not have money problems, celebrities have their own issues to deal with – which is why they need to turn to Ali for life coaching in the first place!

So, remember that until you are happy in yourself, losing weight will never make a real difference to your life. You'll just be a miserable thin person instead of a miserable plumper person! But if instead you choose to be grateful for what you've got, and know that you *deserve it all and more*, you'll exude happiness from every pore.

Why don't you sing along to your everyday tasks, walk and talk and laugh with energy? You'll soon find you don't need that chocolate fix anymore, or that cake to cheer yourself up, and before you know it you'll be slimmer and fitter – guaranteed! So, sing along to the washing up, whistle to work, chat happily to your friends and neighbours, and live life with enthusiasm … and you'll be so attractive to others that great people and opportunities will seek you out – everyone loves a happy, positive person!

And if you would like some more of my simple, easy Neurostrategy exercises to help you along, here you are…

Set yourself a time limit of 15 minutes for this exercise.

Now write a list of 30 non-achievement-related great things about yourself. Note the 'non-achievement-related' bit: these aren't about what you've *done*, but about what you *are*![8]

If you feel blocked, push through and find something to write – anything! For example, the colour of your eyes, or the fact that you love to dance, or you love your children…

Once you've written 30 great things about yourself, know that you could actually go on and write 100! You know you could…

Now, with 30, or 100, great things about yourself listed, what's not to be grateful for?

Neurostrategists call a vision that we can aspire to with joy a 'compelling future'. A compelling future is what we live for; it's what puts the fuel in our engine! Nelson Mandela's compelling future was a world without apartheid. Your compelling future will be your own, your individual picture of how the sun will rise on your dreams and ambitions! That compelling future is *what you deserve.* So check out this exercise too:

Ask yourself: 'What is my compelling future? How does it look, feel, sound and smell?'

Just go with your first answer, the first positive picture that pops into your mind. Trust that your unconscious mind knows the answer, that your unconscious mind knows the *truth*, because that's the way the unconscious mind works…

Then turn up the volume, brightness and emotion knobs on your picture – your compelling future – so that it becomes even more compelling…

And now take pen and paper and describe your compelling future *in as much detail as you can: the look, feel, sounds, smells…* Take 10–15 minutes to do it. Time yourself – that way you'll be getting as much of that valuable detail as possible by forcing yourself to write it all down with a deadline. The more detail in your vision of your compelling future, the better you're programming your unconscious mind to achieve it! Remember that the unconscious mind cannot differentiate between what's real and what's vividly imagined. So write down that great, real, vividly imagined picture of your compelling future right now!

When you've done that, ask yourself: 'Can I imagine myself being the happy, confident and energetic person I deserve to be *right now*? I *am* my compelling future *right now!*'

If you are wondering about that statement, think for a moment. Is there really a difference between the 'you' in your compelling future, and the 'you' in the here and now? It's still you, and you are your own raw material, aren't you? No one else can change *for* you, can they?

You're all you need to create your own compelling future ... so do it!

Remember that any limitations you impose are just that – limitations imposed by *you*. And when you're grateful for all the great things you *do* have, and know you deserve all that and more, there really are no limitations!

So, make a habit of visualizing yourself and your good fortune every day in your mind, taking time to be grateful for all the good in your life. If you find this hard, just try picturing yourself living in Afghanistan or Gaza or North Korea or Zimbabwe, or any of the world's other troubled areas instead, and you'll realize just how much you *do* have – like enough food, safety, freedom from persecution, education for your children, medical and dental treatment for you and your family, a job, an income, relative prosperity, and so on! What a gift!

And the more you acknowledge you *deserve* your good fortune, the more gratitude you will feel – and the more you will have to be grateful for.

Lastly, remember that *slimy*, *sticky*, *gooey*, *crunchy* and *oily* calories do *not* make us happier or blow our problems out of the window. All they do is increase the size of our problems – by increasing the size of our hips and thighs and tummies, and clogging our brains and our ability to feel happy and carefree. Many of these 'feel-good' foods also clog our arteries, which can potentially reduce our life-span… So turn to yourself and ask:

'Does my compelling future want anything to do with gunk?!'
and:

'Do I want to meet my compelling future? How long am I going to keep it waiting for me?!'

Key Points to Remember
- Live with a sense of perspective. Our problems are often pretty minimal compared to those of many in this world.
- Being thin or rich will never make you happy if that's all you aim for in life. Remember you are rich and healthy already in so many ways.
- Instead of dwelling on your worries and bad fortune, be aware of your *good* fortune every day, give thanks for it and be grateful.
- The more we are grateful for the great things in our lives and know we deserve them, the more we will attract them.

- Remember that you deserve all the great opportunities the world has to offer and more.
- Vow to give back to the world the happiness and joy it has given you.
- Create your own compelling future.

Key Number Five

Fill Up your Life!

Just like smoking, eating when you're not hungry gives your body and mind something to do. It's a way of keeping occupied, dealing with boredom or coping with emotions we'd prefer not to confront directly. Hands up, those who are familiar with snacking as a 'displacement activity'!

Eating's undeniably a pleasurable way of taking time out and has been providing us with comfort right from birth: babies cry when they're hungry, children are given 'treats' for being good, and as adults we naturally associate food with good company and good times.

But eating is a *choice*. If you choose to eat rather than getting to grips with a task or facing up to problems or emotions, guess what – you're taking an easy way out! *An easy way out and an easy way to put on weight!*

There's nothing wrong with enjoying food, nothing wrong with a treat, nothing wrong with the pleasure of savouring delicious food that will nurture us body and soul! But to get the most enjoyment out of food, we have to respect it. My father likes to say, 'Too much of anything is good for nothing.' Enjoying healthy food that will nurture us, in the right context and quantity, with respect for its health-giving qualities – *that's* what balanced eating is all about. But when you eat to fill up your life, it isn't about balance. It isn't about respecting yourself – it's about *dis*respecting yourself. It isn't about respecting the nurturing attributes of food either. Do you want to know what eating to fill up your life is? It's *abuse.*

Yes. Abuse! Let me say it again: *abuse!* Eating for comfort, or out of boredom, or to anaesthetize emotions is no different from substance abuse – just more socially acceptable! It's still abuse – abuse of your health, of the life-giving attributes of food, of your time, of your energy, of your life. It's filling up your life with misdirected energy. It's channelling precious

29

energy into eating when your body does not need it. Not only can that energy not be employed elsewhere to add value to your life, but you'll find that *indigestion, cravings* and *becoming overweight* are your body's reaction to being abused.

When you eat to procrastinate, what are you doing? Are you making *an excuse?* Think about it carefully. What could eating be an excuse for? An excuse for not taking action? (Are you lazy or a coward?) An excuse for not being brave and facing up to emotions? (Will eating make the problem disappear?) An excuse for not moving forward in life? (What are you waiting for? What are you afraid of?)

Ask yourself, '*Why am I filling up my life with excuses? Excuses are for wimps!*'

Happily, you've got a choice. Think back to the times when you were so full of energy and plans that snacking was the last thing on your mind! Can you remember a time it happened to you? Can you remember a *specific* time when you didn't eat until you felt true physical hunger, when you didn't think of food until your stomach felt really empty? Can you remember a time you were so excited, so full of life, that food was the last thing on your mind? Bet you didn't need an excuse then, while you felt so full up with the moment – full to the brim with emotions, full of joy! It's not a coincidence that people lose interest in eating when they fall in love, or move house, or get a new job!

So, let's do a little exercise...

Read this exercise through until you are familiar with it and then commit to following the instructions precisely and seriously. You can do this exercise *now* and daily.

Relax now ... and think back in time.

Can you remember a time when you were so excited that eating didn't matter to you? Take your time and remember it.

Can you remember a *specific* time? Take your time and remember it clearly.

Now go right back to that time. Float down into your body... See what you saw, hear what you heard and feel *all the feelings* of being *so* totally full of great emotions that eating didn't matter...

Are you there? Now take those feelings and amplify them...

And *really feel what you felt as strongly as you can! Crank up all the knobs and really feel those feelings ... now.*

Now take those feelings and put them in a special place in your heart and mind, so that when you need them, they will be there for you.

Do it now. That's right.

And when you feel the desire to eat when you don't need to, you can access those feelings to fill you up instead. You've put them in a special place so that they'll be there whenever you need them.

So, why do you think people lose a lot of weight when they fall in love, or move house, or get a new job? It's simple – they're spending all their time doing something *much more exciting* than snacking, and suddenly there's no need to comfort eat out of boredom, simply no time to spend opening the fridge and thinking about food! If this makes you want to open the fridge straight away because your life simply *isn't* that exciting, then *stop!* Picture yourself closing the fridge with a bang before you even look inside – and then walk away defiantly. That's right! Now read on.

Ask yourself, do you need to fill up your stomach or do you need to fill up your … your *what*? That's right, *your life!* So, *fill up your life instead!* Take up a hobby, go out, spend time with friends, meet new people, plan a holiday, refurbish your house – this is an opportunity to do things you really enjoy doing but have maybe felt too lazy or too sorry for your sorry ass to do recently! Lucky you! You have the opportunity finally to get stuck into those wonderful things you've always wanted to do! This is your opportunity to change your life!

Seriously, those who get out there and do fun things are slimmer than those who mooch around the house being couch potatoes. If you don't believe me, look around you. I know you can find examples in your own life that prove my point exactly. If all the excitement you get is sticking around opening the fridge and dreaming of the next meal – and honestly, how *pitiful* is that? – well, are you really surprised that you're overweight?

It's all very well knowing this, of course, but what about when you are near that plate of freshly baked chocolate chip cookies with the crunchy, gooey bits? Now is your mouth watering? It's nothing to do with hunger, or you'd be sitting eating a meal right now instead of reading this page! Your mouth is watering because of conditioning, anticipation and neurological programming.[9] Learn to tell the difference and you'll never fight a craving again!

I'll help you to know the difference later, but in the meantime here's an exercise that will help to you beat cravings…

Please write down 20 strategies – yes, 20 strategies – to beat eating when you're not hungry. Do it now. Do it carefully! This exercise could change your life. So push yourself. Push yourself to the full 20. If you can write down 20 strategies, you can lose all the weight you want!

Now take a look at your list.

Did you write something like: 'Get away from [the source of temptation]?'

How about 'Sit down and ask myself what *need* I am trying to address by filling my stomach when I don't require food'?

How about 'Choose to do something much more exciting than eating!'?

How about 'What am I *feeling* that is causing me to want to cover it up by eating?'

These are the kind of strategies that you're looking for. Feel free to use them if you like them, but *always* make sure you *personalize* them.

One of the most valuable lessons in life is to learn to confront your feelings instead of covering them up. Covering a grazed knee with a sticking plaster is great. But covering up feelings isn't great. They'll only find other, worse, ways of being heard.

'Now you're fat, how about listening to me?' says Pain when comfort eating has been a sticking plaster for too long.

'Now you're exhausted and ill, how about listening to me?' says Tiredness when you've been burning the candle at both ends, fuelling up with sugary snacks and coffee.

'Now you've had a breakdown, how about listening to me?' say Negative Emotions that have been ignored again and again.

If your problem is eating instead of facing up to uncomfortable emotions or situations which you really need to work through, it's simple: you need to work through those emotions. It's your *number one priority*.

That may not sound like much fun, and it will feel uncomfortable at first, but will soon become easier. It will help if you are physically getting out there and doing other activities to increase your sense of positivity at the same time: a new hobby, a bit of sport or simply walking. Be busy mentally as well as physically and you'll find that weight loss and greater energy will naturally follow.

Here's another exercise to help you to break your conditioning:

Write down 20 occasions when you've snacked or eaten when you weren't hungry. You know when they were – that time you'd had a big meal and still ate cheese and biscuits, or had that after-dinner snack of extra ice-cream, for example. *Be honest with yourself.* The time to be truly honest and take control is *now.* So write them down *now.*

Now write down 20 non-achievement–related great things about yourself. That is 20 things about how you *are*, not what you've achieved. 'I love to dance!' for example, or 'I have nice-coloured eyes!' Think of all the great things other people say about you. Think what your mum or best friend would say about you.

You did this in Key number four, you say? Why should you do it again? Am I dopey? Have I forgotten? No, I haven't! This is a great exercise and can only do you *more and more good* each time you do it! Trust me: I'm a trained, certified and qualified Neurostrategist! So, just do it, please, once more, because it's good for you.

Then take a few minutes to review what you've written down.

And say to yourself: *'Look at all the great qualities I have! Do I need to eat food I don't require?'*

Now review the list once more.

And say to yourself: *'Looking at this list of great things about myself, how am I going to fill up my life now?'*

Take 10 or 15 minutes to answer this last question. Answer it in writing.

Keep the list of great things about yourself and twice a day, morning and evening, read it and then read how you're going to fill up your life. Consider this a prescription for weight loss. Take it as seriously as a medical prescription. *Because great people don't need food to make their lives great!*

Key Points to Remember
- Being busy all day and only coming into contact with food at mealtimes is the best training for eating only when you are hungry – the best way to become slim and stay slim!
- Be interested in activities, ventures and hobbies other than food and you will find that snacking, comfort eating and eating out of boredom are no longer what you want to do.
- Beware of using eating as a 'displacement activity' to avoid confronting tasks or emotions which you find uncomfortable. Work through the emotions and tackle the tasks, and simply by taking action you'll feel energized and relieved!
- Review your list of great qualities and how you are going to fill up your life twice a day, morning and evening. Treat it as a weight-loss prescription!

Key Number Six

Lighten Up!

In Key number one we talked about how habits can be used to our advantage. We're all learning how we can profit hugely from good habits. But what if a 'good' habit becomes an obsession? What happens then? Consider the difference between the profitable habit of saving 20 per cent of everything you earn and how Charles Dickens' Scrooge behaves. He isn't praised by anyone for his obsessive saving – he's become a figure of ridicule and a by-word for the worst form of miserly meanness!

Obsessions are particularly destructive because they are a frustrated (and frustrating) over-exertion of brain power. What we colloquially call 'brain power' is actually nothing more or less than *energy*. Remember that:

Where, to *what* and especially *how* you apply your energy determines your life.

Let me say that again:

Where, to *what* and especially *how* you apply your energy determines your life.

Now write that down. It's possibly the most important thing you will ever learn:

> *'Where, to what and especially how I apply my energy determines my life.'*

This could be the key to making your dreams come true.

How you apply your energy is particularly important. Watch long-distance runners: do they push themselves to the limit, veins bulging, the minute the starting gun sounds? No! They pace themselves. Habits are about pacing yourself, building on specific thoughts and actions day after day after day. Obsession, on the other hand, is about running yourself into the ground in one burst – an unlikely winner!

Keith Cunningham, a remarkable businessman and success teacher, hits the nail on the head when he says: 'Ordinary things done consistently produce extraordinary results!'[10] Write that one down too. It will serve you well. You can even stick it up on your fridge...

No one ever lost weight both permanently and healthily by obsessing about it. Granted, you might lose weight short term, but all that thinking about food will convince your unconscious mind that you need it as much as you think about it. Obsession with food can also bring on eating disorders, which potentially lead to very serious health problems, both mental and physical.

So, it follows that *the less you think about food, the more you free up your brain power to be productive and successful.* You are freeing up what I call 'working memory' to allow it to create productive thoughts that can make you successful, rich and more besides...

We seek out what we think about most, so if we think all the time about how we're trying *not* to snack, what do you think the result will be?

A basic presupposition of Neurostrategy is that the unconscious mind does not process negatives. So if I say to you, 'Don't think of a blue elephant,' what do you think of? Exactly.

So, you attract what you *do* want by thinking about it, and you attract what you *don't* want by thinking about it!

This is really important, so ... write it down!

> You attract what you *do* want by thinking about it, and you attract what you *don't* want by thinking about it.

You are realizing now that your thoughts determine your actions. It's also the *quantity* of thoughts that makes a difference. Obsession crowds out your mind and leaves little space for anything else.

Several philosophies – Buddhism, Zen Buddhism, *feng shui*, for example – are built around the principles of harmony and balance. Choose balance and you'll free up important brain power to create abundance in your life. In Eastern philosophy, balance is the key to health, wealth, long life and abundance!

Exaggerated behaviour around food also serves to confuse our metabolic rate (the process whereby our food is converted either into working energy or stored as fat). Our metabolic rate is influenced by our muscle mass, caloric intake and level of exercise and the type of food we eat. By going from one extreme to another – eating too much or too little, binge eating or yo-yo-dieting – we convince our body to store more food as fat. We also upset the weight-control centre located in the brain (the 'ponderostat') which prejudices future attempts to reach a stable weight. In addition, this imbalance leaves us unable to have a healthy relationship with what should serve to nourish us.

Food is, after all, simply a fuel, albeit an enjoyable one, and should not be the object of obsession or hatred. Just imagine how disrespectful and uncompassionate it would appear to a mother on the African continent whose children are slowly dying of starvation to be told that some people in the rich, abundant West have an uneasy relationship with food. We should instead be grateful for our daily nourishment, because if anyone in this world has the right to be obsessed with food, it is precisely that African mother, not you or me. Take a quiet, truthful moment to acknowledge this fact.

Ask yourself:

'How will I take my focus off food and use my energy productively to help transform my life and that of others?'

Take pen and paper and write this question down now.

And now write down 10 answers. Your unconscious mind always has the answer, so let your instinct guide your pen. You may surprise yourself – in a good way!

Will you channel the energy you use to obsess about food into a new, exciting, opportunity – into a new hobby or career, or your family or friendships? When will you start? What do you think will happen?

Put your focus on improving another area of your life and you will lose weight too.

Don't seek out food – seek out success instead!

Key Points to Remember
- *Where*, to *what* and especially *how* you apply your energy determines your life.
- Obsession is a waste of energy – energy that could be used productively elsewhere.
- Obsession with food can lead to serious complications such as eating disorders at one extreme and weight gain or obesity at the other.
- Exaggerated behaviour around food also confuses our metabolic rate. By binge eating or yo-yo-dieting, our bodies are convinced to store more food as fat.
- Balance is the key to success. This means balance in thought as well as action.
- Be careful what you think about, because that's what you'll attract.
- Don't seek out food – seek out success instead!

Key Number Seven

The Good Guilt Trip!

Guilt is a very strong warning signal that we're behaving in a way that doesn't suit us, a sign that we've violated our own moral standards and need to repair our self-esteem and pride. But when we allow ourselves to *listen* to our feelings of guilt, we can act on them to change our behaviour.

Interpreting guilt in this way is very powerful. Psychologists call this 'healthy' or 'appropriate' guilt, because it's being used productively to bring change.

Ask yourself, 'What do I feel guilty about and what do I need to change?'

Then *listen* to the answer!

Write it down now.

Pride, shame, guilt and embarrassment are what psychologists call 'self-conscious emotions' which can be used to self-monitor and control behaviour.[11] So use these emotions to best advantage. Your unconscious mind *knows* what is good for you. Acting immediately on a feeling of guilt to make a positive change is a real boost to your pride and self-esteem. Leveraging guilt in this way makes you stronger.

Whatever you do, don't *misuse* guilt, for example: 'I've eaten two chocolate biscuits and I feel so guilty about it, I might as well finish off the rest of the packet!' This creates a negative spiral that's *very* dangerous for the figure and for self-esteem. So, keep PP (not *that* type!) on hand at all times – that's *Positive Pride*! I call it 'behaving with elegance'.

Sadly, we often ignore guilt's warning signal and continue with our unproductive behaviour until it's pointed out by someone else. Then we are embarrassed into changing. This is because pride is the flip side of guilt, so it's not until our pride is hurt that we felt guilty 'enough' to make a change!

Think of a time when someone really criticized you. Were you shocked and angry because your pride was hurt? But did you realize later (after you'd calmed down!) that there was more than an element of truth in what was being said? Did you feel ashamed and guilty and then decide to make a change? Despite the embarrassment, was it, in hindsight, a positive experience?

When we're conscious of how we appear to others, we behave differently – which is why people behave (and eat!) differently in McDonald's than in a Michelin-starred restaurant with silver service.

You can be your own 'fly on the wall' at any time. Seeing yourself as others see you requires honesty and a dose of courage, but it empowers you. Note that it's *not* about basing your actions on other people's opinions or judgements, but about having the objectivity to be your own judge and jury to incentivize your own positive changes.

Objectivity allows us to move away from being self-centred. It enables us to evaluate our own actions and make positive changes.

When the ex-Spice Girls singer Geri Halliwell wrote her second autobiography and admitted that she'd scavenged through George Michael's refuse bins at Christmas to find leftover cake to binge on, I'm sure I wasn't the only person to cringe! She was very brave to admit it to the world. By 'naming' and 'shaming' her bulimia, Geri was making a powerful statement of intent. She was refusing to live in denial any longer. By being objective about her eating disorder, she could move beyond guilt and proudly commit to change.

Bulimia is a guilt-driven disorder. Geri chose the flip-side, pride, instead. She's wasn't exactly proud to have behaved the way she did, but she's definitely proud to have fought her illness and won! Today Geri is happy and a healthy slim weight.

When we acknowledge our guilt, we can start taking targeted and specific action to make a change. Then we can be proud of our progress!

Every day our unconscious mind is bombarded with a huge amount of data. We have to filter a lot of this or we'd quite simply go mad! Our thoughts, our models of the world, even our identities are the result of how we've processed all the information around us, the result of what we've deleted, distorted and generalized – which means *our* reality is not always the whole truth. (Have you seen the movie *The Matrix*?)

When we have too tight a grip on a problem, sometimes the problem seems indistinguishable from ourselves. Here are examples of what 'I am my problem' could mean:

'I am fat,' says one person.

'I am an alcoholic,' says another.

'I am depressed,' says a third.

Their problems are being assumed into their identities. Their problems are *becoming* their identity! Does that seem right to you?

Do you think Geri Halliwell *was* a bulimic? Or was she much more than that? Whatever you think of her (and I admire her for being driven and plucky and creative!), she actually wasn't a bulimic and never was.

Furthermore, if you say you *are* something, where's the urgent need for change? When negative behaviour becomes your identity, in a way you've accepted it and learned to live with it. The guilt that forces change is no longer there. The objectivity that causes self-evaluation is no longer there. If it's your identity, does that mean there's now an excuse for it...?

So, if you think you are fat, *stop right there!* The minute you realize that being fat is *not* your identity, you free yourself up to choose to be slim instead: you change your identity!

And that's why guilt can be important: because it can *encourage a shift in identity.*

Guilt can be a great incentive for positive change!

In Neurostrategy we encourage people to float into their future 15 minutes after the successful completion of an event, where it has worked out even better than hoped. This allows them to 'disassociate' from – detach from, or view objectively – any event and gain a position of learning and strength. In this way, they can also detach from any event which didn't work out as planned and look at it objectively in terms of the knowledge and experience gained.

Check out these affirmations:
- 'I am concerned about my weight problem.'
- 'I am not concerned about my weight problem.'
- 'There is no such thing as being concerned about my weight problem.'
- 'I am not concerned about my weight problem, as there is no such problem!'

And how about these:
- 'I will not be concerned about my weight problem.'
- 'I will not have a weight problem.'
- 'There will not be a weight problem for me to be concerned about!'

Now, which sentences sound and feel the freest and most effortless to you? Shall I hazard a guess? How about:
- 'I am not concerned about my weight problem, as there is no such problem!'
- 'There will not be a weight problem for me to be concerned about!'

Notice that in each of the sentences there's no association between you and the problem. And if it's no longer yours, then it has no business with you, has it?!

One of the most important things we can ever learn is that we are not our problems, we adopt them. Trouble is, adopting fatness or drunkenness or depression or any disorder is like adopting a wolf into a flock of lambs. Turn to yourself and say, *'Bad idea!'*

As far as Geri Halliwell was concerned, painting such a graphic picture of herself at her lowest point meant that she had to disassociate from the behaviour. That way she gained the objectivity to take action to throw out the bad 'wolf'. If you no longer *are* your behaviour, you can pinpoint it more easily – it's no longer hiding behind the cracks and crevices of ego and pride and denial. You can identify it, take action, grab it by the neck and throw it out! Whoosh! Out it goes, gone forever!

In the film *The Private Lives of Pippa Lee*, starring Robin Wright Penn, the heroine, Pippa, catches herself on her home CCTV indulging in secret midnight binges. What a wake-up call! In front of the fridge spooning in the ice-cream – how embarrassing, how undignified! I watched this film on a plane and although I never really was one to 'midnight feast' in any case, it put me off even the smallest after-dinner snack forever!

If you've ever suffered from compulsive eating, like Pippa, what you need to do is acknowledge the hungry wolf. Acknowledge the problem. Then you can step back, be objective and plan how to overcome it.

Of course you don't actually need to film yourself in real life (that would be a *different* type of reality TV!) – though if you did, the shame might cure you forever! The good news is, you can create a visualization in your mind to access every time you feel you're about to slip into unwanted behaviour.

To do this, let's use a version of a technique to displace negative behaviour and establish positive behaviour. You're going to run a little movie in your head of yourself at your most unguarded, undignified, shameful dietary worst. You know the type of occasion: cream cakes at midnight or something similar – feel free to substitute your very own guilty secret! You are actually going to access the way the memory is 'wired' into your unconscious mind and then switch the wiring to make a positive change. This is the 'miracle' of Neurostrategy!

So … can you think of a time when you ate compulsively, or binged, or overate?

Can you think of a specific time?

Go back to that time now … go right back to that time… Float down into your body. See what you saw, hear what you heard and feel all the feelings you felt … when you ate compulsively... Are you there?

Now, take this picture and shrink it down and put it down to one side...

Done?

Right! Have a little shake of your shoulders before going on to the next bit!

Now you're going to 'change the movie': you're going to take out the movie reel you've just been viewing and run a *new* version where you behave with balance and moderation, doing what's right for your health and figure and fitness. You're going to *behave with control and elegance,* treating both the food and yourself with the respect you're due.

If you can't think of a time when you did this, please imagine the ideal situation of you resisting temptation and exaggeration and eating with balance, moderation and respect.

Can you think of (or imagine) a time when you ate with control and elegance?

Can you think of a specific time?

Go back to that time now ... go right back to that time... Float down into your body. See what you saw, hear what you heard and feel all the feelings you felt when you ate with control and elegance... Are you there?

Now imagine all those feelings are on a dial and *crank it up even more! Crank it up as far as the volume and brightness and colour will go. Make the sights, sounds and feelings as strong and intense as they can be. And then some!*

Now make the version of you being balanced and elegant *even bigger and brighter and louder and bring it closer towards you...*

And now it's so big and bright and light and loud that you're rising up into the air above, together with this new, healthy image, holding it close to you ... while the previous one of you 'misbehaving' is left down below and fades away ... fades further and further away into the distance below ... eventually fading out completely way down below ... gone ... gone ... gone. It's gone and there's nothing left of that old behaviour.

Now have a little stretch and shake out your shoulders.

Repeat the exercise several times, doing it faster and faster each time. The brain does not learn slowly, so speed is necessary to cement the learning. The more you repeat, the more you are rewiring your brain for positive change! You can also visualize your old behaviour as a punctured grey balloon in the fog, collapsed and sinking lower and lower and faster and faster and becoming more and more indistinct until it fades from view forever. Meanwhile, the new behaviour can be a nice big sparkling hot-air balloon and you can be in it, calmly and steadily rising up and feeling bright and beautiful and on top of the world!

You can do this exercise as often as you want. Do it every time you feel temptation knocking at your door. You can also link your movie with other occasions you aren't proud of, seeing each image as part of a string of beads.[12] Then you can replace the old ugly beads with new sparkling beads, each one representing a positive change you're making in your behaviour and life!

While you are mastering a new way of behaving, remember that eating slowly and deliberately is not just elegant and well-mannered (and stops you looking like a gluttonous swine!), but also *helps* you to eat less, lose weight and stay slimmer!

Want to know a bit more about these Neurostrategy exercises? This process of visualizing behaviour you want to stop and replacing it with new positive behaviour is called a '"swish" pattern' or 'pattern interrupt'. Effectively, the new pattern replaces, or 'interrupts', the old pattern of behaviour. You can even make a 'swish' sound out loud to confirm the switch, or say a loud 'Yes!'

This pattern is a basic neuro-linguistic programming technique. NLP was first developed in the US in the early 1970s by Richard Bandler (who taught it to me) and John Grinder, who studied the psychology and behaviour used by highly successful people ('behavioural modelling'). Today it is used all around the globe by millions of people to improve their performance in such varied fields as management, sales, marketing and PR, therapy (including phobia removal), personal development, sport and entertainment, politics, government and even the military! It's used by multi-national companies to train staff and by Olympic athletes, celebrities, politicians and royalty. Paul McKenna and Ali Campbell are two famous NLP masters in the UK. In the US, there are Tony Robbins and Steve Linder. Steve, who works extensively with Tony, is my teacher and is developing cutting-edge Neurostrategy techniques which go beyond traditional NLP, many of which I am sharing with you in this book. These are the *world's most powerful techniques for behavioural change*!

Why is visualization absolutely key in NLP and Neurostrategy? Because people who focus on and *move towards* what they *want* are more successful than people who focus on what they *don't want*. And visualizing *what you want* is the key to getting it.

Now take pen and paper and write it down:

'Visualizing what I want is the key to getting it.'

So, use these visualizations to your advantage, then use your pride – the flip side of guilt – to help you keep feeling proud of yourself!

Key Points to Remember
- Guilt is a warning sign that we are not behaving in our best interest. We can use this 'self-conscious' emotion to make positive changes.
- Objectivity allows us to move away from being self-centred. It enables us to evaluate our own behaviour.
- We are not our problems, we adopt them.
- We can use visualization to replace negative behaviour with positive behaviour.
- When we identify negative behaviour, we can take action, grab it by the neck and throw it out! Whoosh! Out it goes! Gone forever!

Key Number Eight

The Bad Guilt Trip!

In the previous Key, we talked about *Positive Pride* and using guilt productively to identify where we needed to make a change. But there's also *bad guilt*. Bad guilt stops us enjoying experiences and feelings and creates low self-esteem.

The minute you feel guilty as you hide behind the fridge or cupboard door, cramming in that biscuit when you 'know you shouldn't', you are on the road to perdition, my friend... For a start, you aren't enjoying the crammed-in biscuit at all! So you need another, so you can enjoy that one instead, and before you know it, you're in a vicious cycle of bingeing on the whole packet and swearing to yourself you'll go back on the diet tomorrow!

Of course it's not the biscuits' fault. It's *your* feelings of guilt that allow you to love/hate them. You are also loving and hating yourself. Love and hate aren't the key to moderation, however, and moderation is the key to reaching and maintaining your ideal weight. One biscuit never harmed anyone, nor did one chip, crisp or square of chocolate... Not all at once, of course!

So, *never* eat with guilt. If you feel that sneaky sense of foreboding creeping up on you, put away the biscuit barrel. Don't contaminate what should be a delicious experience with guilt. Guilt plus biscuit still equals calories and you haven't even enjoyed it – what a waste!

Guilt also makes people eat more: they're actually comfort eating because the guilt is making them feel so bad! It's a vicious cycle! But once you're aware of it, you can change it.

Here are four rules to follow:

- *Eat with pleasure.*
  Make it a conscious choice to enjoy your food. Choose your food carefully and be happy with your decision. By loving your food, you're loving and nurturing yourself. You're treating both the food and yourself with respect. So, enjoy eating!

- *Eat in moderation.*
  Eating in moderation will prevent any recurrence of guilt. And if you eat without guilt, moderation comes naturally – you won't

need extra biscuits to make yourself feel better.

- *Befriend your food.*
  When you feel guilty about eating, you are demonizing your food. Calling food 'naughty' also has this effect. Choose healthy, nurturing food you can feel good about.

- *Treat yourself.*
  You can allow yourself a treat and thoroughly *enjoy* it, without guilt. That way you will automatically require less to be satisfied. A treat eaten with joy and in moderation never harmed anyone – in fact it's a message that you're happy and willing to treat yourself well and with respect!

When I was working on this book, I had one biscuit every afternoon and one small piece of chocolate every morning – no more, no less. I ate sensibly the rest of the time. I really enjoyed and embraced these treats, and I still lost a couple of pounds in the process (being busy does help you to eat less)! But if you eat the whole packet of biscuits at once, there's no way you'll burn up that energy – it'll go straight onto your hips!

To choose to eat without guilt is empowering. You are making your own choices and you are happy with them. People comfort eat when they feel guilty and trapped and powerless, but if you are empowered and balanced, then to be honest, you don't need to get your kicks from a cream cake!

Key Points to Remember
- Never eat with guilt. Don't contaminate what should be a delicious experience.
- Guilt makes people eat more: they're comfort eating because the guilt is making them feel so bad! But once you're aware of this, you can change it.
- If you eat without guilt, moderation comes naturally. To choose to eat without guilt is empowering.
- Follow the four rules:
- Eat with pleasure.
- Eat in moderation.
- Befriend your food.
- Treat yourself.

Key Number Nine

Get Motive-ated!

If you suspect you're eating when you're not physically hungry, then please do question your motives. Be pro-active and acknowledge the problem, and then, like all first-rate investigators, get to the root of the matter.

Here is a list of 'hunger motives' to help you get to the bottom of why you're having that craving…

Thirst

Ask yourself first, is it *thirst*? Try drinking a large glass of water and then wait a few moments. Are you still hungry? Our body very often mistakes hunger for thirst.

It's intensely important to keep hydrated: water not only regulates body temperature, it also improves digestion, helps to transport nutrients through the body and aids in the elimination of waste matter and toxins. Most importantly, dehydration impairs your mood and your cognitive performance, i.e. your ability to think and act clearly.[13]

Boredom

Or are you craving food out of *boredom*? If it *is* boredom, ask yourself whether snacking on sugary foods will turn your life into an adventure or just make you fat and miserable. People who feel depressed about their weight are less likely to get out and do interesting things, which in turn makes them even more bored. So, do you think that eating to relieve boredom is really a good idea?

If a little voice tells you (it's your unconscious mind speaking!) that you might be eating out of boredom, don't kid yourself otherwise and don't make excuses! Acknowledge the *real* reason for suddenly feeling peckish and thank your intuition.

Note that genuine hunger doesn't suddenly arrive, but gradually creeps up on you. Any sudden or random sensation of hunger isn't the real deal: it's greed!

Before reaching out to food to ring the changes or fill a need, how about *being productive*? This means using your time in a valuable way to make your life better. *Do you want to spend your time becoming fat and unfulfilled or healthy, wealthy and slim?*

At the very least, why not take a walk to the nearest newsagent's and buy a newspaper to read? Feeding your brain is by far preferable to feeding your body unnecessarily, and if feeding the intellect is not for you, how about a magazine or novel? (However, do beware of glossy magazines which encourage comparing yourself to artificially slim celebrities: pointless and damaging.)

A feeling of 'need' does not have to be filled with food. Instead, fill it with novelty, excitement or joy. How about learning new skills that will increase your power and success in life instead of filling your stomach?

What you need is not food, it's fulfilment. Don't kid yourself.

If what you crave is a *change* — for the better — then make that change! You change nothing by eating, except your shape! Make a change in your surroundings: go out and visit a friend, make a phone call, go for a jog, take a bath or shower (to relax or energize yourself) or indulge in a creative hobby. The aim is to keep yourself occupied and give yourself a boost. I would guard against watching TV, as television is passive entertainment and rife with adverts designed to get you salivating, so it's not the best choice of distraction! A DVD or movie is also passive entertainment, but if it works for you, then fine, as long as you omit the popcorn! Do try to fill your life with interesting pursuits which won't make an ounce of difference to your waistline, and the more active or energizing, the better!

Now take pen and paper and write down:

> *'My "need" is not for food to fill me up, it's for fulfilment. I will get fulfilment not by abusing my time but by spending it getting a richer life. And I will get a richer life not by eating but by doing!'*

Repeat this as often as you feel a craving to eat when you're not hungry. If you act on it every time, I guarantee the results. Hands down!

Excitement

Food has been used for millennia to celebrate. But enjoying food at a party is one thing and treating yourself to chocolate cake alone in your kitchen because you're excited about something is another!

Excitement is not an excuse to overeat or eat when you aren't genuinely hungry, even if the butterflies in your stomach are (supposedly) making you feel all weak and woozy!
Don't eat when you're excited – will you still be excited when you find you've put on weight?

Emotional Reasons

If you have a tendency to eat for *emotional reasons* rather than out of natural hunger, then how about *stopping and thinking* before opening the fridge or cupboard?
Overeating, drinking too much alcohol, smoking and abusing drugs (prescriptive medicines as well as narcotics) are all attempts to anaesthetize uncomfortable emotions – but the effect's only temporary! Do you think that getting fat/drunk/stoned (or even in trouble with the law) will make the sad event or difficult situation go away? Or do you think it can only add to it by bringing *more problems* to your life?
The best way to help yourself when you're experiencing uncomfortable emotions is to help others or spend time with friends and loved ones. This raises self-esteem and releases the feel-good hormones associated with caring.
Steve Linder asserts that all 'negative' emotions can be boiled down to five: *anger, sadness, fear, hurt* and *guilt*, in that order. (Anger, for example, often masks sadness, and so on down the line.) But remember that these feelings are only 'negative' if you fight them. If, instead, you acknowledge them and their reason for existing, you can find the silver lining. Ask yourself, 'What is this emotion teaching me? What have I learned from the events that preceded the emotion?'
However tragic an event may be, there is always something to learn from it – about yourself most of all and how strong and resilient you really are.

Gaps

Other sorts of *gaps* in your life may manifest themselves as a feeling of craving or hunger. Of course there probably *is* a craving or hunger there, but it just *isn't to do with food!*
There was a time in my life when I was feeling creatively frustrated, and when I'd feel that sensation of achingly searching for something, I'd open the fridge and search for a snack. (Oh, naughty me – see, we're all human!)

I felt a gap of sorts and instinctively turned to food to fill it. I was putting on weight until I acknowledged the problem, made changes in my life to solve the issue and promptly lost the weight. I'm much more careful now to question my motives if I have unexplained feelings of hunger.

If you do this too, you will find it will have the significant effect of changing your behaviour for the better. So, when will you start?

How about this? When you feel a GAP in your life, use the acronym: *Go Acknowledge Pain.*

Acknowledge what you are feeling and take five minutes to write it down.

Then take another five to ten minutes to write a 'Gap Buster' list! This is a list of all the positive actions you are going to take to close the gap. (Tip: Eating food is not one of them!)

Repeat to yourself: *'Eating food will not help me get rid of nasty gaps in my life!'*

Now take pen and paper and write it down.

Further on the subject of gaps, many people who are overweight have a love gap in their lives: they're searching for a partner or companionship and eat to fill the space where they feel a relationship 'should' be. Of course it can become a vicious cycle, because being overweight makes it more difficult for some people to have the confidence to get out there and meet new people. The whole process is self-defeating!

What do you think they should be doing instead of eating? What do you think they should be focusing on - instead of concentrating on what they *haven't* got? Remember that you attract what you think of most, so if you think of what you *haven't* got, then...?

What's the answer? Think of what you do want and do what you can to attract it! Lose weight, get fit, get gorgeous and get out there – and lots of potential love interests will come running. Once you start to shine, others will be attracted to your glow!

Energy creates energy, and this is especially true in relationships, whatever stage of the process you're at. Once you're on the journey to success, your sense of increasing self-confidence will be appealing and engaging to others. Now turn to yourself and say: *'That's me: energetic, motivated and self-confident!'*

Anger or Frustration

If you are eating out of *anger* or *frustration*, again realize that compulsive eating will only compound the problem by making you feel fat and out of control, and that's on top of what is already causing you to be upset and imbalanced! So, *don't do it!* Instead, aim to find a constructive way out of the anger or frustration and a solution to the problem that caused it in the first place (or, if there's no solution, simply be philosophical and accept what you can't change). Anger and frustration are debilitating and freeze you into inaction like the brake on a car. Release the anger lever to free yourself up to move on!

Alternatively, you can rise elegantly above your feelings by putting them into perspective. (Floating above an issue is a really useful visualization.) Don't sweat the small stuff! Don't be a coward and get hot under the collar! Anger is a lack of control. So get real and don't make it worse by overeating! Do you think being out of control is going to get you anywhere or anything?

Instead, *be productive!*

It's Expected of You

Sometimes, overeating is a risk because you feel it's *expected of you*. This is a special problem in those cultures where 'Eat, eat!' is a rallying cry. What to do? You need to save face – *and* save your shape!

So, take stock of yourself, feel *strong* and clever, and make sure you show the hosts you're enjoying the food immensely. Just don't let them notice you've got tricks up your sleeve: you're eating at *half the speed, taking plenty of sips of water* and *making conversation instead of eating*! (This is also an effective trick with wine at those parties where the glass is always being topped up if, like me, you fall over after one glass of white!)

When asked if you want seconds, choose healthy options like vegetables, and politely decline the unhealthier ones. People notice acceptance before refusal, so your choice of green beans over roast potatoes is unlikely to offend.

My friend Dr Isaac Jones calls people who 'encourage' others to eat 'food pushers'. In fact, food pushers can exert such pressure that you risk overeating out of frustration, let alone politeness!

There are two types of food pusher. One has a hidden agenda, wanting you to eat too much out of jealousy or envy that you're slimmer than they are or losing weight when they wish they were instead. This is the more dangerous type. Ignore their nasty tactics and let them know you're not going to be manipulated.

The other type has to be treated with consideration. Many female relatives can fall into this category. They see their role as the provider of food as part of an emotional relationship. If you refuse food, it's like refusing their love! So, tread carefully. Praise the food immensely, while choosing larger amounts of healthier food and tiny amounts of the rest. If you have to refuse something, explain that you usually love it, but you're trying to lose a spot of weight and their loving support would really mean a lot to you. Remember they want to nurture you and show their love by offering food and are craving appreciation and praise in return.

Reversing the roles – serving them and making sure they have enough food, or helping to serve others and clear the table, pour drinks, etc. – can also work by taking the focus off what you are eating and still gives the hostess the consideration she craves!

Instinctive Reasons

Mums often finish off their children's uneaten food for *instinctive* reasons – show me one mother who hasn't had the urge! This is a natural response engendered during millennia, as in the past the best tidbits were kept for the young, so couldn't be wasted.

Understanding that this is a hard habit to break, I simply serve myself less of my own portion, knowing I'll finish at least some of the children's meal in addition to mine. In this way I end up eating the same amount but not fighting with nature!

Displacement Activity

Displacement activity – finding something to do in order to 'displace' another task – is another common reason for feeling hungry when there's no true physical requirement to eat. We all know it better as taking a tea or coffee break. A nice 'cuppa' with a chocolate biscuit somehow seems to happen just when you know you've got that important task to finish off or when hunky James from Accounts walks towards the staff kitchen! Before you know it, 15 or 20 minutes have passed. Result? You still haven't started on that urgent job, and not only that, you've just stuck that biscuit right onto your hips or belly. (And James won't like that!) Make sure it's a lesson learned for next time!

Key Points to Remember
- If you suspect you're eating when you're not physically hungry, stop and question this sudden urge to eat.
- Look for 'hunger motives':
  o Are you *thirsty* instead?
  o Are you using food to relieve *boredom*?
  o Are you rewarding *excitement*?
  o Are you wanting to comfort yourself with food, using it as an *emotional* crux — or are you craving a natural anaesthetic or a temporary stimulant?
  o Do you have a *gap* in your life you're attempting to fill with food?
  o Are you eating out of *anger* or *frustration*?
  o Is overeating *expected* of you at certain occasions?
  o Are you overeating *instinctively* — finishing up the kids' food, for example?
  o Are you using food as a *displacement activity*?
- Distract yourself from the temptation to eat by taking action and doing something positive for your mood and self-esteem.
- Work on solving the underlying issues.
- You *will* break this pattern. When will you start?

Key Number Ten

Can the Self-Control

It's basic: when you deprive yourself of enjoyment, the end result is frustration and denial. It's human. But humans don't like frustration and denial and the result is overcompensation, a 'flip reaction'. This is one reason why crash diets don't work.

If you enjoy food, you won't enjoy denying yourself. Full-stop. Period.

You may find yourself daydreaming constantly about what's forbidden! But the more you think about it, the more you'll move *towards it* instead of away from it. Remember, you attract what you *don't want* by thinking about it. And you can think about it way too much — the very fact that a certain type of food is 'forbidden' can lead to it becoming an obsession, causing unnatural hunger feelings and episodes of overeating or bingeing to compensate. And overeating or bingeing results in weight gain, so, in a nutshell, dieting can make you fat!

Turn to yourself and repeat: 'Dieting makes me fat! Balance makes me skinny!'

Now write it down:

'Dieting makes me fat! Balance makes me skinny!'

On the subject of dieting, have you heard of the yo-yo dieter? He wound himself up! Sorry, I couldn't resist that one... But we've all heard of someone who restricts what they eat and loses weight, then overcompensates by overeating everything they missed during the diet, puts the weight back on and the vicious cycle starts again. (That's not anybody you know *personally*, is it? Not from now on, it isn't!)

Denial, obsession and bingeing can also be symptoms of serious eating disorders, like anorexia and bulimia nervosa. These require serious medical intervention, as they can be fatal. If you know, or think you know, someone who's suffering from an eating disorder, please do seek the advice of a qualified health professional before it's too late.

So, how about *enjoying* eating healthily and losing weight? Is it possible?

Yes, it is, but there are some things to watch out for. First of all, beware of substitutes. 'Diet' foods – low-fat and so-called 'light' versions of treats like crisps, cakes and biscuits, often with artificial additives in place of the fat and sugar – are formulated to dupe your body into thinking it's still being given its treats, but do you think your body believes it for a moment? 'Diet' versions of food can increase cravings, because your body expects the same degree of satisfaction it normally gets from sugar and fat and is *not* satisfied with alternatives. Come on, after millennia don't you think your body's cleverer than that? Food substitutes are simply ... substitutes. They can't pass for the real thing.

Also, it's not sustainable to eat artificial 'garbage'. Artificial sweeteners, additives, trans-fats, hydrogenated fats and other chemicals *are* garbage (you can find out more in *'The Toxicity Trap'*, see Chapter 5). Remember, if you eat garbage, you will *feel* like garbage. And what will you *look* like? So, can the bad food substitutes if you want to can the obsessive cravings!

To satisfy a craving, allow yourself a small piece of what you fancy. That's a *small* piece! And don't forget to increase your energy expenditure by doing a little sport or being active so that you burn it off.

To achieve balanced eating without the need for excessive self-control, continue to eat what you enjoy but in small portions. Stop when you're full and always concentrate on enjoying the taste, texture and aroma of your food. I call this 'conscious eating'. If you've been used to overeating, this strategy alone should be enough to help you to lose your excess weight. Here are three simple rules for conscious eating:

1. Eat consciously and in small portions.
2. Don't eat when you're not hungry.
3. Concentrate on fully enjoying the taste, texture and aroma of your food.

Do you think that people of a healthy weight don't love food? *Wrong!* Most love it, but they also know how to eat with balance, avoid cravings and enjoy occasional treats.

The more you respect yourself and your nutritional requirements, and the more you acknowledge that food's life-giving properties are also worthy of respect, the more likely you are to be slim and fit.

What's the secret to treating food with respect? Savour your food with gratitude and attention. Eat it in the right amounts, at the right times, and make the right choices. No extremes, no love–hate relationship with food.

Those who banish or forbid food (not you, of course) just create unnecessary resentment, tension and stress for themselves. They're grappling on a slippery slope that isn't sustainable. Sooner or later they'll slide right back down, 'Wheeee!', to that wobbly tummy!

What about you? Well, now you're committed to treating your body, your health and your food with respect and making this a sustainable long-term strategy, guess what? Before you know it, your progress will feel truly effortless. Just picture that! Because progress isn't about 'self-control' – it's about putting new strategies in place to make progress effortless!

Key Points to Remember

- If you enjoy food, you won't enjoy denying yourself. The result will be overcompensation.
- If you forbid yourself something, it can become an obsession and you will attract it.
- Instead, follow the three rules for conscious eating:
  1. Eat consciously and in small portions.
  2. Don't eat when you're not hungry.
  3. Concentrate on fully enjoying the taste, texture and aroma of your food.
- Treat food with resect: eat it in the right amounts, at the right times, and make the right choices. No extremes, no love–hate relationship with food.
- Progress isn't about 'self-control' – it's about putting new strategies in place to make progress effortless!

Key Number Eleven

Have a Game Plan

It's fine to enjoy good food and good wine – even tasty desserts! In fact, it's absolutely necessary to eat your food with the greatest of enjoyment so that your body and mind are satisfied. When they are, you'll be free of cravings, feelings of deprivation, compulsive eating, overeating and an unhealthy love–hate relationship with food. You'll find that you appreciate food for its ability to nurture you, strengthen your health and contribute to optimum vitality and energy.

As you know by now, moderation is the key. So, if you're on holiday or in party season, be wise and have what I call a 'game plan': either factor in extra exercise or make sure that *balance* is involved. We all like to relax and enjoy good food on holiday without the stress of counting the calories or being too faddy. But if you're going to get slim and stay slim, you'll have to get wise and stay wise.

Now take pen and paper and write it down:

'To get slim and stay slim, I'm going to get wise and stay wise.'

When you're used to overeating, your body becomes unable to differentiate between natural hunger cues and greed. This becomes a vicious cycle: the more you overeat, the more you're programming your body – as well as your mind – to overeat.

Also, when you make *excuses* for overeating – whether it's a special occasion, a holiday, or you feel bored, or sad, or frustrated, or unloved – you'll put on weight. Remember, *excuses are for wimps.*

Turn to yourself and say, *'Excuses are for wimps! Excuses mean I'm not honest with myself. Excuses mean failure, not success!'*

A big 'excuse' for overeating are those times of the year when there's a lot of eating going on – festive seasons or festival days, or parties, or holiday mode, when you're feeling extra relaxed and wanting to overindulge that little bit. It's fine to enjoy the good things in life, but it's also important to enjoy them in moderation. Remember the 2 Rs: *realistic* and *reasonable*. Eat *reasonably* and be *realistic* about the consequences of overindulging. Follow times of plenty with times of moderation. If you have a dessert at lunch, for example, have a light dinner of lean protein and vegetables or salad.

Ask yourself, *'How much is it worth to me to maintain my weight?'*

And if your aim is to lose weight, ask yourself, *'How much is it worth to me to maintain my weight loss?'*

Remember that every bite of food that you don't need will just go straight onto your hips, or your love handles, or paunch! As Steve Linder says, 'There's no such thing as an inconsequential bite!'

So, ponder for a moment and ask yourself, *'What have been the consequences for me of too many inconsequential bites? And sips?'*

Now ask yourself: *'When will I start making every bite and every sip count? Is now a good time to start?'*

Remember, excess energy consumed and not burnt off means excess weight. It's a simple equation and doesn't stop being relevant on holiday!

Use my 'Divide up and Rule over' concept: *divide up* your food consumption and spread it over a longer length of time. This means what you don't eat today, you can always eat tomorrow. You can also use wise combinations to make sure you don't exceed your energy requirements. This is how to *rule over* how much, when and what you eat.

For example, if you've eaten a large main meal but fancy a dessert, why not have that dessert tomorrow, and then don't eat it with a large main meal but with a salad or lightly cooked lean protein? Or if you're at a restaurant, choose a light starter instead of a main meal, which balances out the dessert. Remember, however, that desserts shouldn't be everyday treats if you want to maintain a healthy shape and avoid the trap of sugar cravings!

Choosing to eat certain foods tomorrow instead of today has to part of your game plan from now on if you are to maintain a slim weight and the fitness that comes with it. This means not serving yourself everything every day from your holiday buffet! Try something one day and something else the next. It has been proved scientifically that more variety means we consume more.[14]

The same goes for parties – you can always ask the host to pack a slice of cake to take home because you've eaten enough. I do it all the time and no one ever minds – in fact other people often gratefully follow suit! The same at restaurants: don't feel you have to finish it all up if you've over-ordered, just ask for a 'doggy bag' 'to go'! All bar the most expensive restaurants are used to this by now. In the most expensive ones, the portions are so small you won't find food left over anyway!

Take control – have a game plan and choose *when*, *where* and *what* to eat!

Key Points to Remember
- The key to a healthy, slim and happy life is *balance*. Balance times of indulgence with moderation, cutting back when necessary to redress the balance.
- There is no such thing as an inconsequential bite or sip.
- Eat *reasonably* and be *realistic* about the consequences.
- *Divide up* your food consumption and *rule over* greed.
- Take control – have a game plan and choose *when*, *where* and *what* to eat.

Key Number Twelve

Energy Creates More Energy!

Enjoying physical fitness can be incredibly powerful, unlocking great energy. It's a fact, folks! Being honed and toned encourages a natural 'get up and go'. Even thinking of the word 'fit' gives energy and 'buzz'! But often people who are overweight feel heavy, and feeling heavy means tending toward inaction and laziness, either for physical or psychological reasons.

But guess what? Overweight people actually burn up *more* calories than slim people simply because they're moving a greater mass around! OK, granted that to move a greater mass requires a greater effort – but the payback in calorie-burning is greater too!

When the overweight person feels that exercise is going to take a lot of effort, just that thought could be enough to exhaust them! They're not realizing that, wow, when they actually start to exercise they'll be burning up a whole load of calories to kick-start the weight loss. The extra load is actually like lifting extra weights at the gym!

But it's the old chicken and the egg scenario: you need energy in the first place to create the desire for the gym, the park, the swimming pool, even climbing the stairs! How can you get it?

You know what? You can get energy while still in your armchair just by visualizing yourself being fitter. Would you like to try it out?

Now if you would like to, just go ahead and see if you can close your eyes. And I wonder if you can sit quietly and remember a time when you were totally energized... Can you remember a specific time?

Go back to that time now ... go right back to that time... Float down into your body and see what you saw, hear what you heard, and feel all the feelings of being totally energized...

And now take all those sights, sounds and feelings of being totally energized and make them brighter, louder, stronger and more intense.

And now make them 100 times brighter, louder, stronger and more intense!

And now squeeze them into your right fist – there! That's right.

And now squeeze them even tighter into your right fist – there! That's great! You're doing fantastic!

And now squeeze them as tight as you possibly can! There.

When you are ready, slowly let go and come back into the room.

And whenever you need those feelings of being totally energetic, simply squeeze your right fist. That's right! They'll be right there for you. Those feelings of being totally energetic are right there for you.[15]

A Case Study

A client, Anne, 26, who works in the media, was somewhat overweight, but since her mother's mastectomy due to breast cancer, she was determined to get fit and healthy. To commit to change in a big way, she signed up for a sponsored ten-kilometre run, raising money for cancer research, a cause that now meant a lot to her personally.

She started off by adopting a healthy nutrition regime and subscribed to the gym, initially under the gentle guidance of a personal trainer, aware that *change + action = progress.*

To make the challenge more *realistic* and *reasonable,* Anne also visualized herself running the course every day and walked the route several times, picturing herself in her mind's eye passing the finishing point.

Whenever she felt nervous about a new challenge, for example increasing the length of her practice runs or her workout time, or cutting out sugar from her diet in order to eliminate cravings for snacks, she said to herself, 'I may not be ready *yet,* but I will be ready when I *am!*'

She also worked with *commitment, consistency* and *congruency.* Day by day she worked out and ate healthily, and day by day the results were there to egg her on as she lost pounds and gained muscle and felt her endurance increasing week by week.

Now she's completed the run and collected the sponsorship. She proudly wears the T-shirt while pounding the streets training for her next run. 'I've got the bug!' she laughs.

Anne may not have been an energetic and fit individual when she started out, but she saw herself as one, even if only in her mind's eye. And guess what? Her unconscious mind believed it *even before* she'd achieved the end result! Remember, the unconscious mind doesn't differentiate between what is real and what is vividly imagined.

Anne aligned her self-image and identity with the change which losing weight was to bring and this gave a message to her unconscious mind to produce the results. What if she'd been unable to imagine herself as passing that finishing line? What do you think would have happened then?

Napoleon Hill, author of the legendary book *Think and Grow Rich,* said, 'Whatever the mind of man can conceive and believe, it can achieve. Thoughts are things! And powerful things at that, when mixed with definiteness of purpose and burning desire…'[16]

Now take pen and paper and write it down:

> *'Whatever the mind of man can conceive and believe, it can achieve. Thoughts are things! And powerful things at that, when mixed with definiteness of purpose and burning desire…'*

Anne also asked herself several questions which can help *you* to achieve your goals. Here they are:

- 'How much do I want to achieve this?'
- 'What does it mean to me?'
- 'What will I lose if I fail to achieve this?'
- 'How will I feel if I don't achieve this?'
- 'What will I gain by achieving this?'
- 'How will I feel when I achieve this?'
- 'What's hanging in the balance?' (Beliefs or values? Family or friends? Health and fitness? Love? Etc.)

Now work on answering these questions for yourself. Sit quietly for 20 minutes (time yourself) and write down as much detail as you can. Trust that your unconscious mind has all the answers, so let the pen flow across the paper without thinking too much.

Like Anne, you too can find the engine to power your dream! And remember that energy and fitness are infectious. Some of Anne's friends were originally sceptical about her dream, but now they're thinking about getting fit themselves and maybe joining her on a run too!

As Anne puts it, in true media style, 'I took a pot-shot at my dream with an enormous cannon ball!'

Key Points to Remember
- Enjoying physical fitness can unlock great energy.
- Overweight individuals have more body mass to move, so they actually burn more calories than slim people for the same amount of exercise.
- Exercise becomes effortless once you attach it to a dream or ambition.
- Visualize yourself being energized and it will translate into physical energy.
- Take a pot-shot at the target of your ambition with an enormous cannon ball!

Key Number Thirteen

Link to 'Higher' Stuff

Psychologists have linked self-affirmation – thinking about values that are important to us – with the ability to 'structure information and focus on the big picture'.[17] What does this actually mean? Put simply, when we repeatedly link our goals to what we value most, we increase our motivation exponentially. It's like being powered forward by a jet-propelled rocket!

So, when you want to lose weight, linking that goal to something you value way *beyond* the weight loss will be much more effective than concentrating on the pain of foregoing chocolate muffins.

Consider the following statements – do any of them apply to you?
- 'If I take immediate, consistent and sustainable action to lose weight, I will be able to take a more active role in my children's upbringing by being able to play sport and undertake other activities with them.'
- 'If I take immediate, consistent and sustainable action to lose weight, I will live longer by reducing the health risks posed by being overweight.'

- 'If I take immediate, consistent and sustainable action to lose weight, I will be more able to accomplish other goals and ambitions because I won't be taking up valuable time and energy worrying about being overweight.'
- 'If I take immediate, consistent and sustainable action to lose weight, I will take the focus away from how unattractive I feel and will be able to concentrate on creating meaningful relationships.'
- 'If I take immediate, consistent and sustainable action to lose weight, I will set an example of health and energy to my children and family.'
- 'If I take immediate, consistent and sustainable action to lose weight, I will be fitter and have more energy to pursue my career successfully.'
- 'If I take immediate, consistent and sustainable action to lose weight, I will be healthier and more energetic and better able to serve my clients.'
- 'If I take immediate, consistent and sustainable action to lose weight, I will be in a better position to conceive and give birth to a healthy baby without health complications.'
- 'If I take immediate and consistent action to lose weight, I will prove to myself that I can take action and achieve results and I can use this confidence to achieve other aims in life!'

My friend Priyanka Patel's higher purpose was to love and serve others by becoming a paramedic. She had to lose weight to pass the physical, but once she was sure of her purpose in life, not eating her favourite cakes was no longer a sacrifice! She went from a size 22 (US 16) to a 12 (US 6) in little over a year.

Another client – let's call her June – was unhappy, overweight and unhealthy. She was so dependent on comfort eating that she kept a chocolate bar beside her bed. One day the telephone beside the chocolate bar on the bedside table rang: a close relative was bravely fighting terminal cancer. June immediately felt ashamed, realizing her relative could no longer choose to improve her life or her health, but that she could. In that transformational moment, she resolved to lose weight and stop bingeing. She thought how petty it was to struggle with the urge to eat a chocolate bar in bed when a loved one was struggling simply to stay alive. In that moment she vowed to accept the precious gift of life and health and honour it. She'd no longer die through obesity. With this higher purpose in mind, she went down to a size 8 (US 2), gained incredible energy and fitness, and converted her entire family to a healthier diet and lifestyle in the process!

Having a higher purpose certainly revs up our motivation! Then it helps us *stay* motivated and go all the way to success. It puts the small discomforts we may be going through during the process into perspective.

Another way of putting it is 'delayed gratification', which means delaying a small amount of pleasure now in order to gain a far greater reward in the future. More on this later.

So, what might be your higher purpose? You'll find it's something absolutely crucially important and non-negotiable to you as an individual. Looking at your values will give you a clue. Here are some examples of values which might inspire a higher purpose (in alphabetical order):

- family
- freedom
- friendship
- health and fitness
- honesty and integrity
- legacy
- life and death
- love
- personal growth
- serving others
- spirituality or God

Now we're going to do a little exercise to clarify your values, OK?

Write down what's important to you about the values above, one by one.

Now, can you think of any *other* values that are meaningful to you? Time yourself and take five minutes to come up with any others that are particularly relevant to you. (Remember to write down the details of what's really important to you about the additional values you've added as well.)

Now do a double check to make sure all the values you've written down really mean a lot to you. They have to resonate really strongly with you. They have to be powerful enough to push you to seek success and stay the course.

You should now have a definitive list of values you feel are important in your life right now. (Our hierarchy of values is subject to adjustment and modification as we move through life.)

Next, please number the values according to their importance to you.

What's the most important? What's next? Etc.

Then rewrite your list of values in the new order on a clean sheet of paper.

Now choose the one which resonates most with you – which hopefully is number 1.

Can you remember a time when you were totally motivated in the context of [value]? Can you remember a specific time? As you remember the time … what was the last thing you felt just before you were totally motivated?

This exercise gives you clarity over what's most important in your life. And now that you're aware of your values, you can use them as drivers to hook up your goals to – that's a lot of horsepower!

It'll also amaze you when you realize that what you thought were negative states or emotions can actually be powerful drivers too. Let me explain. It may be that the *last thing* you felt just before you were totally motivated was something like frustration, discomfort or pain. Certainly, in my life, I make great leaps and bounds just after I've felt frustrated with where I am! It may be the same for you. How great is it to discover that your negative states are simply energy which can be exploited to serve you and help you move up to the next level of achievement in life?!

Now write down how your values link into your goals and vice versa. For example, I linked my goal of finishing this book with my values of 'Serving others' and 'Leaving a legacy', as well as helping to contribute financially so that my family can have the lifestyle I wish for them.

To understand how you might tie in your higher purpose to your goal of losing weight, ask yourself:

> 'What will I lose by losing weight?'
> 'What will I gain by losing weight?'
> 'What does losing weight mean to me?'
> 'What and who will be affected if I don't lose weight?'
> 'What and who will benefit from my losing weight?'

And finally ask yourself:

> 'When will I start using my higher purpose in life to fuel my goals and ambitions?'

Key Points to Remember
- Having a higher purpose behind our goals provides us with much more powerful motivation.
- So link your goals to something which is really important and non-negotiable for you as an individual.

Key Number Fourteen

Visualize, Visualize, Visualize…

We already know that by visualizing what we want to achieve we are giving a clear directive to our unconscious mind to take the path of least resistance to it. So, let's understand the unconscious mind a little better…

Our unconscious mind stores, organizes, represses and resolves memories. It makes associations and learns quickly. It is the domain of the emotions and it controls and maintains perceptions. It generates, stores, distributes and transmits energy, maintains instincts and generates habits, enjoys serving, and runs and preserves the body.

Crucially, it responds to symbols and doesn't process negatives, so whether a sentence is positive or negative, the picture we see in our mind (our 'internal representation') is still the same. For example, what's the first image in your mind when you read: 'I must not eat cakes'? You eating cakes, right?!

It therefore stands to reason that if we are trying to harness the power of the mind, it is more efficient to use images rather than words, and positives rather than negatives. If someone wrote 100 labels saying: 'I must not eat cakes' and stuck them around the house, how effective do you think that would be in getting them not to think of (or eat!) cakes?

On the other hand, what's the first image in your mind when you think: 'I'm going to be slim and fit'? You being slim and fit! So visualizing yourself as slim and fit and telling yourself you're on the path to being slim and fit very soon is a powerful technique!

Picturing your goals in broad, colourful detail, including all the feelings, sights, sounds and even aromas, serves to 'fix' these images into the unconscious, where they become 'real' in the same way that memories or dreams are real. The unconscious mind does not differentiate between reality and vivid imagination, and is able to *create* reality simply from the images it receives.

Sportspeople, especially at Olympic level, as already noted, use visualization all the time. Studies have been conducted to measure the increase in performance it can generate.[18] In one study on creative visualization, for example, Russian scientists compared four groups of Olympic athletes with training schedules split differently between physical and mental training:

- *Group 1:* 100 per cent physical training
- *Group 2:* 75 per cent physical training with 25 per cent mental training
- *Group 3:* 50 per cent physical training with 50 per cent mental training
- *Group 4:* 25 per cent physical training with 75 per cent mental training
- Group 4, whose training encompassed a high 75 per cent of mental training, were the top performers![19]

As Albert Einstein said, 'Imagination is greater than knowledge.' Isn't it amazing that every creation and work of art, every accomplishment, was first conceived as an image in someone's mind? How wonderful to realize, as you are reading this, that the mental images you construct as a blueprint can, now you understand this, become your reality in the same way as the architect's sketch becomes bricks and mortar!

Let's start to use the power of visualization quite simply by getting used to thinking permanently in the positive. Instead of 'I feel fat' (and your mind's eye will see that image and reinforce it, so take an eraser and rub it out until it has disappeared from the surface of the page and your mind, please), think, 'This is what I look like at my ideal weight!' and 'I can see myself slim and I *am* seeing myself slim!' Picture it now as you are looking at it. Now step into the picture. And now you *are* the picture – and can feel all the feelings associated with being your slim self!

If you think, 'I must not eat crisps,' your mind will imagine eating crisps. If that just happened, take a big dustbin full of rotting maggots, throw the crisps into it, suppress the nausea, wave away the stench and ... do you still want to reach out for a crisp now?

Instead, turn now towards an orchard which is in full bloom and think, 'Yum, I love all that tasty fruit, the satisfying sweetness of those super blueberries and the aromatic crunch of this red apple fresh from the tree,' and you will find you desire the fruit more and more, more and more. That's *right*!

If you're interested in reading more about how to use the language of the mind to consistently achieve your desired outcomes through neuro-linguistic programming, there are plenty of books out there and you'll find several listed in the resources in the back of this book.

Remember, you *are* what you imagine yourself to be and *can become* what you imagine yourself to be!

Key Points to Remember
- The unconscious mind cannot differentiate between reality and vivid imagination and is able to create reality from the images it receives.
- You can start to use the power of visualization quite simply by getting used to thinking permanently in the positive.
- You are what you imagine yourself to be and can become what you imagine yourself to be!

Key Number Fifteen

Don't Keep Up with the Joneses!

Nowadays, our increasingly materialistic society is obsessed with closing the gap between the 'haves' and the 'have-nots'. The most popular TV talent shows offer 15 minutes of fame, and reality shows provide insights into the world of the rich and famous so the man on the street can feel even more awestruck – or resentful! Whatever happened to what my mother and grandmother used to tell me: 'Be content with what you've got. What you've got is quite a lot!'?

This modern obsession with wealth and celebrity produces often envy – wanting what others have and you don't: physique, lifestyle, possessions, skills, talents, beauty and so on. Envy is secretly – or not so secretly – resenting others for their good fortune. It's about concentrating on what you don't have in relation to what other people do have. But do you remember what happens when you concentrate on what you *don't* have? You attract more of the same!

It's no wonder that envy is the fastest route to being dissatisfied, unhappy and depressed: with your income, weight, appearance, environment, marriage, job – anything!

The Tenth Commandment of the Bible foresaw this danger thousands of years ago:

> 'Thou shalt not covet thy neighbour's house, thou shalt not covet thy neighbour's wife, nor his manservant, nor his maidservant, nor his ox, nor his ass, nor anything that is his.'

And in the Book of Luke (12:15) it is written: 'Take heed, and beware of all covetousness; for a man's life does not consist of his possessions.'

Saint Thomas Aquinas noted envy was 'sorrow for another's good'[20] – the opposite of charity.

Buddhism states that desire for earthly things will tie us to the wheel of reincarnation: the Third Nobel Truth of Buddha suggests that if one can eliminate desire or attachment, one can eliminate suffering.

In the Muslim faith, Allah orders believers to seek refuge from: 'the evil of the envier when he envies'.[21] 'Indeed envy eats up good deeds just as fire consumes firewood.'[22]

Hindu scriptures warn: 'Among the profuse precious things a man may acquire, none surpasses a nature free from envy toward all.'[23]

And the Yoruba people of Africa (all 28 million of them!) have a saying: 'Covetousness is the father of disease.'[24]

In the fable attributed to Aesop, the goose that laid the golden egg was killed out of greed: 'Much wants more, and loses all.'

Various proverbs also highlight the inherent dangers in envy, for example the British 'The grass is always greener on the other side of the fence', the Arab 'Every ambitious man is a captive and every covetous one a pauper', the German 'Envy eats nothing but its own heart', the Bulgarian 'Other people's eggs have two yolks' and the Mexican 'Envious persons never compliment, they only swallow.'

That's an awful lot of wisdom crossing cultures, countries and centuries! It seems that no matter the religion or background, wise people agree on why defining ourselves by what we *own* – instead of what we *are*, what we *do* and how we *act* – is so unhealthy. By the way, do you agree that celebrities should be excused drug abuse, tax evasion and insulting behaviour?

Envy turns values upside down and prevents compassion and sharing. Most dangerous of all, it prevents us reaching our own true potential. Envy is dangerous. It can hold us back from achieving anything!

Do you remember that *how you use your energy determines your life*? When you are envious, your energy isn't being harnessed productively. Instead, it's being burnt away in bitterness and ingratitude, anxiety and stress. By focusing on *other people*, you lose sight of your own self and ignore your own resources and potential!

Envy is limiting: it keeps you thinking about how you don't measure up and feeling bitter about it (whether you acknowledge that bitterness or not). It reinforces a state of 'lack' and inferiority. It makes it really hard to proceed from a position of knowing that life is *abundant*...

Envy focuses the mind on the end goal in the wrong kind of way: on *other* people having what you want! But crucial for results-based thinking is the ability to see *your own self* in a position of success. By constantly instructing the unconscious mind that other people are successful and you are not, you are focusing on your limitations and your inadequacies and erecting mental barriers to hold yourself back.

Remember, what you visualize becomes your reality!

There's also a crucial difference between focusing on what you want and focusing on how to get there. The first is an abstract desire. But the second is the road map! Just wanting something is static – there's no action or movement. Once you have a plan of *how* to achieve something, you release a lot of positive energy which will propel you in the right direction.

I've coming from a place of experience here, folks! I spent years seeing the gap between myself and women who were taller, slimmer and more elegant (I conveniently ignored the ones who weren't!) My boyfriend once called me 'short and dumpy'. Hearing this, I created a limiting belief in my mind. Years later, someone else I cared about told me I was 'simply gorgeous' and worked on making me believe it! But I was still basing everything on what *other* people thought…

Do you remember when we talked about living at the cause instead of living at the effect? When you stop focusing on other people, you start understanding your own potential and how to achieve it. You start living at the cause. You stop living at the effect. It's not enough for other people to tell you what or who you are, even if it's *positive*; you have to believe it *yourself*. To believe in your own potential you have to love someone … guess who?!

Take pen and paper and write down who you have to love to understand, realize and reach your own potential.

Now write down a commitment to love that person … write down a commitment to love *yourself!*

This commitment is the key to your success!

We've all been in the envy trap at one time or other. But ask yourself, 'Whose life is it anyway? When am I going to take control? When am I going to start being at cause instead of at effect?'

The trick is to discover how to get to your *own* version of success – and choose to take this route. And then how nice will it be to join those who are fit and slim and healthy (and perhaps wealthy), instead of secretly rejoicing when they put on weight, or make mistakes, or fail (we've all done it in our darkest hour…)?

Don't forget, too, that by envying and resenting others you're creating distance between you and them. You're pushing them away. As a result, you'll never learn from or be part of their world – it's just not possible if you don't accept that world. If you believe that all wealthy, powerful people have cheated their way to the top, for example, you'll never be wealthy or powerful!

Similarly, if you resent other women for being slim and elegant and call them 'skinny bitches', you are simply telling your unconscious mind that all attractive women are ... skinny bitches! And you wouldn't want to be one of those, would you? Could this be why you struggle to lose weight? Ask yourself:

> *'Who am I going to accept into my world today, so I can join their club?'*
>
> *'What place is envy going to have in my life from now on?'*
>
> *Who am I going to respect so that I can respect myself?'*

Key Points to Remember
- Envy is dangerous. It can hold us back from achieving anything!
- To stop being blocked by envy, we have to recognize the value of our own unique qualities.
- When we stop focusing on other people, we start to understand our own potential and how to achieve it.
- We will never learn from or be part of the world of those we push away through envy.
- When we celebrate the ability and success of others, we make it more likely that we'll join them soon!

Key Number Sixteen

What's your *Real* Excuse?

It's story time. Are you sitting comfortably? When you read these stories, ask yourself, 'What stories do I tell *myself*?' and 'What's *my* sob story?'

Once upon a time there was a young intelligent actress who cut herself with a razor where it wouldn't show. The need to feel in control of her pain, any pain, was greater than the pain itself.

Once upon a time there was a business owner with a chain of hairdressing salons who was extremely overweight. She found her self-worth in her business success, as relationships had been a failure. Being overweight gave her an excuse to focus only on what she felt she was good at, and by keeping potential partners at bay not only was she able to devote all her time to her business and become even more successful, but she also avoided exposing herself to inadequacy and possible failure in other areas of life.

Once upon a time there was a young girl from a traditional background who grew up to believe marriage was incompatible with career. A successful entrepreneur, her weight kept her from having to confront a possible mix of the two.

Once upon a time there was an invalid who preferred to be cared for and fussed over by his family than to get better and be independent.

Once upon a time there was a young woman who stayed in an abusive relationship because it reinforced a love–hate and reward–punishment pattern established in her own childhood and gave her a mission in life to 'redeem' her partner. The identity this gave her was worth more than the pain.

Once upon a time there was a man who tolerated his wife's infidelity; it gave him an excuse to be less than honest with her about his business dealings.

Once upon a time there was a serial entrepreneur with a string of failed businesses and marriages. Despite the bankruptcies and divorces, chasing challenges made him feel powerful.

Once upon a time there was a woman who wouldn't lose weight until her husband did, so worried was she about upsetting the 'status quo' in her marriage.

Once upon a time there was a child who continued to misbehave so that she'd continue her sessions with the child psychologist who listened to her and gave her the attention her mother didn't.

All these are true stories: the stories of real-life people who at that point in time were choosing not to make positive changes in their lives because of what is called 'secondary gain' or 'indirect benefit', which means that what appears on the surface to be a problem is actually meeting their needs at a deeper level.

Perhaps one of the most horrific examples of secondary gain is Munchausen's syndrome (or FII, fabricated and induced illness) and Munchausen's syndrome by proxy (factitious disorder). These are tragic disorders in which people 'create the symptoms of illness, either in themselves or in another person ... by pretending to have symptoms that don't ... exist, or by deliberate harm...'[25] The victim may be the perpetrator themselves or, in the case of by proxy, very often a vulnerable dependent such as a child, often the perpetrator's own. The reason for such unnatural behaviour is thought to be an overwhelming and narcissistic need for attention, particularly from doctors, and possibly a desire for abdication of parental responsibility to the medical community.[26]

Addiction is another example of secondary gain. This comes in various guises and can be either extreme – as in abusive relationships, narcotics, alcohol, gambling, etc. – or milder – like 'addiction' to chocolate! Many people reach for an alcoholic drink, a cigarette or a sugar hit because these enable them to relax and feel enjoyment. And alcohol, food, drink and tobacco products (and stronger narcotics, too) all have a double whammy: not only do they have strong associations – parties, celebrations, having fun, freedom, social contact, sexual attractiveness, etc. – but they are also pleasant to consume in themselves!

So, in trying to 'kick a bad habit' the consumer of alcohol, food, etc. is also trying to stop themselves from fulfilling a need, from carrying out behaviour which serves a purpose, from experiencing something which creates a gain! The *immediate pleasure* is perceived as more important than *the long-term risk*.

If you use any substance as a crutch to hold you up, then logically you have a *need* for it. Deciding to 'ban' it won't work unless that need is addressed in some other way.

It's like my gardener, who spends time and effort clearing brambles, only to discover that there's a whole root system underground and that the dreaded stems are going to pop up again in no time! Until that underlying need is confronted and resolved, like the brambles, it will simply resurface time and time again. Once it has been addressed, and met with a positive strategy instead of the addictive substance, there will be a shift in identity from being an addict to being a person who chooses to be healthy. It's this shift that changes behaviour for the long term.

Now please take pen and paper and write this down:
    'When I shift my identity, I change my behaviour sustainably.'

While you have your pen and paper there, here's an exercise for you:

Let's say someone – let's call him John – smokes at parties because if he weren't concentrating on smoking, he'd be standing there at a loss, too shy to approach new people. Stopping smoking may make him feel healthier, even save his life, but it won't do wonders for his self-confidence: in fact it might make things worse, because the certainty which smoking gave him has been taken away. He might not die of lung cancer, but he'll have to confront something much worse – talking to strangers!

What would you suggest he does? Give yourself 10 minutes to write some strategies to help him out.

Done? Now you understand, don't you?

Have you found John another strategy to overcome his shyness?

Say he takes your advice and puts it into practice? What do you think happens now to his need for a cigarette?

And did you know that according to Alan Carr's *The Easy Way to Stop Smoking*, most smokers actually dislike the taste and experience of smoking?

Can you think of how you could apply a similar scenario to someone who impulse eats or comfort eats?

What strategies would you suggest to them?

Done? Now you understand, don't you?

Next let's consider how secondary gain can keep people overweight. Let's use someone – let's call her Jane – for these examples:

- Jane is overweight because she has issues with how she projects her sexuality. (This is common, by the way, with victims of sexual abuse, who may bury their sexuality beneath being overweight because they blame their sexuality for causing the trauma in the first place.)
  Secondary Gain = protection.

- Or perhaps Jane is overweight because she feels she's too shy to approach the opposite sex, or feels undeserving of being approached, so believes that being overweight will guard her from having to confront that scenario.
  Secondary Gain = protection/maintenance of an identity.

- Or perhaps Jane is overweight because in her environment there is a deep-seated disapproval of women being viewed as sexual beings. Being overweight therefore hides sexual attractiveness, prevents a conflict of values and protects the cultural identity from 'contamination'.
  Secondary Gain = certainty/belonging/protection/maintenance of an identity.

In all these examples, there are perceived benefits to being overweight. It protects Jane from the emotional implications of being attractive to others and/or provides the reassurance of not having to question an established identity and enter into unknown territory. So Jane may think she wants to lose weight, but unconsciously there's too much at stake!

Before she can successfully lose weight, she will have to remove the secondary gain and fulfil her needs for protection, certainty and identity in a positive and healthy way.

How about you? Are you constantly trying to make a change for the better but somehow unable to, despite your best efforts? Are you 'self-sabotaging'? Why? Is there a secondary gain there to a greater or even lesser extent?

Write it down.

Ask yourself: 'How is this behaviour serving me? What need is it fulfilling? How can I fulfil this need in a different and healthier way instead?'

Important Note

Please note that in extreme cases of secondary gain, professional help or qualified intervention may be required to get to the root of the problem. Please do not hesitate to seek it as soon as possible. Please note that such situations are beyond my professional scope and liability and the advice given in this book. In the case of abusive or violent relationships, the only solution is to distance yourself as much as possible, before further serious emotional and physical injury can occur.

Now let me tell you another story. Once upon a time there was a homely, working-class, overweight, ordinary middle-aged daughter of a miner and a typist, who'd suffered learning difficulties and been bullied at school. In her own words, her life was 'mundane' and 'routine', and at 48 she'd 'never been married, never been kissed'. She sang on stage in a talent competition and within nine days of the audition, videos of her had been watched over 100 million times. This is the amazing story of Susan Boyle.

Seven short months later she debuted with the number one CD on charts around the globe. In only six weeks, it became 2009's biggest-selling album globally, with nine million copies.[27] In May 2010, she was voted by readers of *Time* magazine as the seventh most influential person in the world – with *five times* more votes than US President Barack Obama.[28]

What do you think would have happened if Susan Boyle had decided that status quo, certainty, maintaining her identity and protecting herself from failure were great reasons to stay at home and had never tried her hand at *Britain's Got Talent*?

Five Powerful Questions to Beat Secondary Gain

Whenever you aim to make a positive change in your life, write down the answers to these five powerful questions.

Why not do it now? Trust your unconscious mind to write down the answers – let the pen move over the paper and write from the heart!

1. 'What have I got to gain or lose by staying *where* I am?'
2. 'What have I got to gain or lose by staying *who* I am?'
3. 'What have I got to lose by making changes? What have I got to gain by *making changes?*'
4. 'What have I got to gain by *shifting my identity?*'
5. 'What have I got to gain by *finding different strategies to fulfil my needs in a positive way that will enable me to progress* in life and achieve my goals?'

Key Points to Remember
- The reason we find it hard to eliminate bad habits is that they may be providing us with secondary gain.
- Examples include staying in an abusive relationship to 'redeem' someone else, smoking to gain confidence around new people or in new situations, overeating because of a fear of being attractive to the opposite sex and eating chocolate because it's easier to relieve boredom that way than make an effort to create a more stimulating life!
- Working on identifying secondary gain can provide the greatest catalyst to change.

- In extreme cases, where there is violence or severe addiction, specialist help may be required. Please do not hesitate to seek it as soon as possible.
- New strategies can be developed using the 'Five Powerful Questions to Beat Secondary Gain' (*see above*).

Key Number Seventeen

Befriend Yourself!

Do you treat your body like some sort of stranger with whom you're uncomfortable? Do you perceive your physical being to be just an outer shell, a wrapping, like an item of clothing? Don't you realize that your body *is* you, one and the same?

Now you realize this, can you in good faith respect your body less than you should? It is your vehicle for life, carrying you around and enabling you to reach great destinations and experience wonderful things. And in life, there is *no* second choice of transport!

Now take pen and paper and write it down:

> *'My body is my primary choice of transport. And there is no second choice!'*

Say your body is the car which takes you through life and your mind the driver – it makes sense that there's no point neglecting either one or the other! Without a car, a driver is redundant, and without a driver, the car remains in the garage. And since our body is such an important vehicle, it deserves special respect, care, maintenance and pride.

In the next Key, we'll talk a bit more about the link between mind and body. But for now, let's look at the body. It is the reflection of what's going on not only consciously, but also in the unconscious mind.

One of the prime directives of the unconscious mind is to run the body and preserve it. It even has a blueprint for perfect health, so if you give it the correct orders to follow, it'll happily engage all its resources to help you to reach that perfect health, in so far as this is genetically feasible.

The brain is connected to the nervous system. It produces hormones and chemical reactions which affect the body directly. This is why body language can 'give us away', as evidenced in lie-detector tests. It's also why we can convince ourselves consciously that we aren't stressed, but nonetheless suffer from stress-related ailments like migraine, eczema and exhaustion. Our body isn't separate from how we feel, or who we think we are: it's the very *reflection* of how we feel and who we are! And the unconscious mind knows just what to do, and knows the truth. We often sadly just don't realize how much we can trust our 'intuition', or how much the 'conscious' mind chatters away, distracting us from listening to the truth, when the answers are there all the time!

Remember that your body is *on your side*. It's just waiting for you to instruct your unconscious mind to take the steps to perfect health. Like a car, if you maintain your body and take responsibility for driving it properly, it will take you far! When will you start – *now*?!

Those who like to say that they're 'a slim person trapped in a fat body' are very, very wrong. Unless we are literally physically disabled, our body doesn't trap us – we trap ourselves! We must all quit making excuses and take responsibility. It's the mind that controls the body.

So, ask yourself, *'When am I going to start to treat my body as the friend it is and work with it to sculpt the healthy, slim body I want and deserve? How long am I going to keep my buddy/body(!) waiting to achieve what it's impatient to achieve?!'*

Key Points to Remember
- Our body is the vehicle which takes us through life and deserves special respect, care, maintenance and pride.
- In life, there is no second choice of transport.
- Our body is waiting for us to instruct our unconscious mind to take the steps towards perfect health.
- We must all quit making excuses and take responsibility. Our mind controls our body and our behaviour, not the other way round.

Key Number Eighteen

A Healthy Mind in a Healthy Body!

The saying 'a healthy mind in a healthy body', *mens sana in corpore sano,* was penned by the Roman poet Juvenal as far back as the late first/early second century ad. So it has been known for centuries that this is something to aim for.

Researchers have confirmed that our physical characteristics affect both how we feel about ourselves and how others judge us. It has been proven that being overweight makes us miserable and, on the flip side of the coin, that exercise and good health improve our state of mind, irrelevant of gender, age, education, income, marital status or religion.[29]

Think being overweight is your personal problem? Think again! The US Centre for Disease Control and Prevention (CDC) estimated in November 2009 that obesity cost the nation $147 billion in medical costs, with diabetes costing $116 billion, and that the percentage of American adults who were obese in 2008 was over 26 per cent.[30] And United Kingdom National Health Information Centre Service statistics for 2010 indicated that the number of people in England having obesity surgery has been rising year on year over the previous decade, with obesity or overweight threatening the health of two thirds of adults and a third of children.[31]

That was several years ago. Since then, things have only got worse.

As these statistics show, the impact of eating too much can be serious and far-reaching. But what most people aren't aware of is that we can banish overeating by working more on the *mind* than on the body, because it is a *symptom*, not a cause. The cause (when medically related or hormonally related conditions are excluded) is more often than not in our mindset.

The relationship between body and mind has been a subject of discussion for centuries by psychologists, philosophers and researchers. Most of us have heard of Pavlov's dog. Pavlov was a Russian researcher whose dog salivated merely on hearing a sound (some say a bell, others a tuning fork) that it related to food. But it's not only dogs who have these reactions. Take a moment and imagine the sensation of an ice-cube in the mouth, or a slice of lemon. What happens to your mouth and lips?

These examples are just the tip of the iceberg. Our mind can be used to exert control over our body to an astounding degree! In Steve Linder's Neurostrategy Master qualification courses, we are able to put students into a state called 'full body catalepsy', whereby the body becomes so rigid through the use of hypnotic suggestion that it can be set between two chairs (neck on one chair, ankles on the other). But this is nothing compared with the feats that sportspeople, ballet dancers and yogis perform all the time, using the power of the unconscious mind to assist them in extreme physical challenges.

For example, in 2002 the *Harvard University Gazette* published an article describing how Tibetan monks entered a state of deep meditation (called *g Tum-mo*) in a room where the temperature was barely above 4^0 centigrade

(40° Fahrenheit). They were covered by sheets soaked in cold water – a situation which served to lower their body temperatures even further and would usually produce uncontrolled shivering and a severe risk to health. But within several hours each monk had dried three sheets with his body heat! Herbert Benson, associate professor of medicine at Harvard Medical School and president of the Mind/Body Medical Institute at Beth Israel Deaconess Medical Center in Boston, noted that:

> 'If such an easy-to-master practice can bring about the remarkable changes we observe ... I want to investigate what advanced forms of meditation can do to help the mind control physical processes once thought to be uncontrollable.'[32]

Researchers also found that monks involved in advanced meditation in Sikkim, India, could lower their metabolism by 64 per cent. Other monks slept on a rocky ledge at an altitude of 15,000 feet in the Himalayas at almost minus 18° Centigrade (0° Fahrenheit), wearing only thin shawls, and slept until dawn with no evidence of feeling the cold. Benson concluded: 'Along with nutrition and exercise, mind/body approaches can be part of self-care practices that could save *millions of dollars annually* in medical costs.'[33]

The monks were a perfect example of cohesion between mind and body. 'Cohesion' can be defined as 'when related parts contribute to a central purpose'. When mind and body are cohesive, the potential to contribute to the central purpose is huge!

Think about this quote : 'Body without mind is brutish; mind without body ... is a running away from our double being.'[34] So perhaps the first focus should be to realize that health and fitness in the body start with health and fitness in the mind.

Key Points to Remember
- Researchers have shown that being overweight does not help us to be happy.
- Taking responsibility for the body starts in the mind.
- We can harness the mind to become slimmer and fitter.
- Health and fitness in the body *start* with health and fitness in the mind.

Key Number Nineteen

Make the Right Decisions!

The quality of your decisions determines the outcome you get. That's true in any area of life. The key to successfully achieving your goals is to make the right decisions at the outset, and then again and again as you make progress along the way.

How do you know what is the right decision? Careful planning will help. It's like when you plan a road trip. You need:

- the *specific details* of where you're going
- an *estimate* of the mileage required and the *timescale*
- a *map* of the territory to put the journey into context and guide you in the right *direction*
- *milestones* or landmarks marked at various stages so you can check you're on the right track
- *flexibility*, in case there's a diversion from the planned route
- *preparation* – all the components of your vehicle well-tuned so that your engine is running smoothly and with maximum efficiency and safety
- *provisions* – petrol in the tank, water to keep you hydrated, money to buy things, a jacket for when it turns chilly, etc.
- *back-up*, in the form of breakdown insurance in case you're stopped in your tracks
- *support* – a co-driver and good map-reader (or GPS) to help you on those long stretches
- *positive energy* – have you ever noticed how a drive seems a lot shorter when you're excited about getting somewhere?

And once you've reached your destination, it's a great idea to:

- *Confirm* you're actually at the right place.
- Take the time to relax a little and *celebrate!*

You knew we weren't just talking about a car journey, didn't you?! It's exactly the same process when we're planning to achieve any goal in life: we're simply progressing through a sequence of well thought-out decisions, each and every one impacting the end result and each and every one propelling us towards that end goal.

Do you think that end goal is separate from our decisions or linked to them all?

That's right – it isn't separate at all…

Now take pen and paper and write it down:

'My end goal is simply the sum of all my decisions.'

When a series of quality decisions comes together to enable an end goal, it suddenly appears effortless. That's simply because the equation of *cause and effect* is a basic rule of the universe. When you tap into this rule with a clear vision and sense of purpose and then support your goal with the right decisions, you'll find that a 'flow' will carry you forward.

Artists, musicians and sportsmen through the ages have talked of this moment of effortless progress. It has also been called the 'creative genie', 'divine inspiration' and 'manifestation'. Whatever it may be, it's all to do with being in the right place and doing the right thing at the right time. And this isn't coincidence, it's because you've made the right decisions along the way!

So, let's talk a little more about the power of decision-making. On the positive side, you have your purpose – that's the big decision you've made to change something for the better! So everything you do should carry you in that direction, right?

Er, not always. Because on the minus side there are those sneaky everyday decisions based on impulsiveness, emotion and instant gratification just waiting to upset the apple cart! These so-called 'snap' decisions are based on emotion, not reason, and might not support your long-term resolve at all. In fact, they risk *sabotaging* your long-term goals.

Can you think of any snap decisions that have sabotaged you in the past? Be honest with yourself. How about writing them down, so you've got them in black and white and you'll be better prepared the next time round?

Here's an example: when you're hungry/tired/bored, you automatically reach for a bagel/biscuit/muffin/chocolate bar to resolve the problem. And it might make you feel better for, let's say, about the time it takes to eat it. Five minutes tops? But the question is, does it *really* make you feel better in the long run, especially if you're trying to lose weight?

We know that most slim people do allow themselves treats from time to time, and that's fine, but what if you make this 'little' decision pretty often? And what if you combine it with other 'little' decisions which don't support your end goal either? Take a look at these decisions made by Jane, someone just like you:

- 'I won't go jogging today. It's raining.' (Monday)
- 'I won't go to the gym today. I'm tired.' (Tuesday)
- 'I'll take the lift instead of the stairs just this once – it's much easier.' (Wednesday)
- 'I'll just have these cookies now and start my diet again tomorrow.' (Thursday)
- 'I'll have a second helping today – I'm wearing baggy clothes.' (Friday)
- 'Leftovers don't have calories…' (Saturday)
- 'It's Sunday – I can pig out on Sunday lunch, hooray!' (Sunday)

Well, that was a productive week then! How much fitter, healthier and slimmer do you think Jane is now?! And what would happen at the end of a month like this, or even a year?

Remember, '*Snap decisions snap your decision!*'

So, what can you do to realize your purpose? It's simple: you support your big decision with a series of smaller decisions. These will be the foundations, helping your dream to rise up tall into reality. Step by step, decision by decision, you are constructing your goal…

Here's a reminder of the process:

- Make a big decision (goal) – to lose weight, for example.
- Understand that this big decision is merely a *sequence of small decisions made day after day, hour after hour, minute after minute.*
- Make the right small decisions repeatedly: no slacking!
- *Make the small decisions based on their future outcomes and* not *their present paybacks.* Ask yourself: 'If I do this, will I still feel I've made the right decision tomorrow?' Imagine that you are reviewing it from the future.
- If you find it hard to predict the outcome of small decisions, *compare them to past decisions* and use that knowledge to make sure you're doing the right thing. For example, if you are tired and want to grab a doughnut, ask yourself how that made you feel the last time you did it. Was the moment of gratification worth it in the long run?
- Turn the tables: place yourself at your end goal and work backwards. You've achieved it, but *how*? Map it out backwards

and then take action forwards! You've given your unconscious mind a flavour of how it feels to be where you want to be, now support it in reaching that destination!

Right, listen up: we're going to do a little exercise.

Take pen and paper. Turn to the list at the beginning of this Key and complete it for your weight-loss journey:

- First you'll write your weight loss and fitness goals in *detail*.
- Then you'll write down the *specifics* of the weight you need to lose and the *time schedule* for losing it.
- Next you're going to jot down any ideas you have of techniques and programmes you might use (which you can add to or clarify as you go along).

And so on.

Make sure your goals are SMART: *specific, measurable, achievable, realistic* and *timely*.

Key Points to Remember

- Be conscious of your decisions and use them to control where you are heading and what you wish to achieve.
- All life-changing and really effective decisions are a series of small daily decisions which support the overall goal.
- Ask yourself how the decisions you make – especially those small ones – will impact what you are trying to achieve.
- If a 'snap decision' won't help your cause – don't do it! *Snap decisions snap your decision!*
- If you are not sure what the outcome of your decision will be, review similar decisions from the past.
- Does what you feel like doing now plug into your greater happiness and well-being in the long term, not just the moment? This is the question to ask yourself in order to make the right decisions.
- Map out the route to your goals and make sure they are SMART!

Key Number Twenty

Are You Concentrating?

Many people have lost touch with how much they should be eating. They overeat because they don't know how to recognize when they're full. In a sense it's not their fault if they're lacking the right information. The good news is it's never too late to learn!

If you have weight to lose, then you no doubt either overeat at times or have done so in the past. If you insist you really don't overeat but still need to lose weight, then are you eating the right foods? Or do you need to move your body more? (Note that if there are medical issues involved, they are beyond the scope of this book and you need to consult a qualified medical practitioner.)

Most people carry excess weight simply because too much energy (in the form of food) is taken in and too little energy (in the form of exercise) expended. It's logical. But if it's such a simple equation, where's the problem? Surely all you have to do is eat less or not eat too much?

'More easily said than done,' I hear some of you mutter! So, how do you go about training your mind and body to eat exactly what's needed?

Have you heard of 'mindfulness'? You might already know that it is an important concept in Buddhist and Hindu philosophy. What does it actually mean?

Put simply, 'mindfulness' means inhabiting the present moment fully, without being distracted. It is the state of being fully aware of *what is*, whether that is a state, an action, an emotion, a sensation or a situation. It means full engagement with all your senses: sight, hearing, feeling, smell, taste.

When you fully *concentrate* on the appearance, texture, aroma and flavour of the food you are eating, and the feelings it produces in you, to the exclusion of all else around you, then, only then, are you eating mindfully. And when you eat mindfully, not only does your body have time to recognize that the volume (bulk) of food you're eating is filling you up physically, but your mind, too, is satisfied and fulfilled by the heightened sensation and the experience of your lovely meal.

If you rush through your food, on the other hand, thinking about your day, what's on TV or what your plans are, even pondering what you're having for dessert while you're still on the main course(!), you're not giving either your body or your mind the time or opportunity to realize you've had enough!

Do this frequently and you'll get fat. Period. Full stop.

In *The End of Overeating: Taking control of the insatiable American appetite*, Dr David Kessler advocates:

> 'Seizing Conscious Control ... a matter of paying attention and recognizing how quickly that attention can be hijacked. It means being mindful of the stimuli that trigger automatic behaviour – a hot slice of pizza, taco chips at a Mexican restaurant, or those aromatic ... cookies – and replacing them with foods that sustain you. Mindfulness also allows you to recognize how entertainment – bustling crowds, loud music, bright lights, or the company of good friends – and the desire to feel better can wrest away your capacity to focus on what you eat. Staying alert to emotional stressors is part of seizing conscious control, so that instead of responding habitually, you're equipped to act defensively.'[35]

Dr Kessler talks about labelling the feelings which might cause you to overeat. In this way, you are being mindful not only of what you are eating but, just as importantly, of what stimuli may *encourage* you to make particular food choices and eat when you do: he calls these 'triggers'.

On the other hand, when you have trained yourself, day after day, meal after meal, to eat slowly, to concentrate on and be 'mindful' of your food, to make food choices which will serve you, to eat only when you are hungry and to stop when you are full., then you should be losing weight and keeping it off in the long term. No diets, no cravings and no regimes – just what nature originally intended! You will find losing weight and keeping it off become effortless!

Mindfulness requires *conscious effort* to truly appreciate food as a bounty and as a blessing. Take a leaf out of the book of the people from the island of Okinawa off the coast of Japan, who are famed for their extraordinary health and longevity (and naturally they keep in shape too): they eat slowly and with care according to their practice of *hara hachi bu*, which literally means 'eat until you're 80 per cent full'. I lived in Japan for three years and – although of course this is a generalization – I observed that the Japanese, certainly the older generation, did eat for the most part mindfully, carefully and slowly. And in general Okinawans consume 10–40 per cent fewer calories than Americans.[36]

You can make this an '80:20' rule to follow. Eat until you are 80 per cent full, then wait 20 minutes for your brain to register that you are satiated. While you eat that 80 per cent, make it well and truly count, and savour each and every mouthful with all your senses. Be mindful, too, of *why* you make the food choices you do and *when* you eat, so that you may 'seize conscious control' of your diet – and your life.

Ask yourself, 'What steps can I take every day to teach myself to be mindful, not just in eating but in all areas of my life?'

Take pen and paper and write down 10 situations in your life where you could be more mindful.

Then write what the real benefit of being more mindful will be, both to you and to those around you. For example, if you are more mindful of what your client or boss is trying to communicate, what could this change represent in your work? And how could being more mindful at home serve to enhance your domestic relationships? How could being more mindful while you make love enhance your sex life? And so on.

Now stretch yourself and write five more. You can do it!

This exercise will transform your life.

Key Points to Remember
- Many people overeat because they don't know how to recognize when they're full.
- Most people carry excess weight simply because too much energy is taken in and too little energy expended.
- You can train your mind and body to eat exactly what's needed by being mindful about your eating.
- Concentrate on all the senses which are being fulfilled by your eating experience: sight, smell, aroma, taste, even sound (as in a crispy apple)…
- When you have trained yourself, day after day, meal after meal, to eat slowly, to concentrate on and be mindful of your food, to make food choices which will serve you, to eat only when you are hungry and to stop when you are full, you will find losing weight and keeping it off become effortless.

- Follow the example of the Okinawans, who are famed for their longevity and health, and stop eating when you are 80 per cent full. Then wait 20 minutes for your brain to register that you are satiated.
- Be mindful, too, of *why* you make the food choices you do and *when* you eat, so that you may 'seize conscious control' of your diet – and your life.
- Ask yourself, 'What steps can I take every day to teach myself to be mindful, not just in eating but in all areas of my life?'

Key Number Twenty-One

Ditch the Distractions

We've just talked about taking time to understand when you're full. But how about the science behind feeling full, or satiated?

There are various scientific explanations as to how, why and when we feel full. First, there's the hypothalamus gland in the brain, which regulates body temperature and food intake. Then there's the *glucostatic* theory, according to which blood sugar levels and the level of glycogen in the liver act as hunger regulators. The *lipostatic* theory talks about fat cells and fat-storing enzymes. And a new *purinegic* theory talks about purine molecules inherent in DNA.

Needless to say, going into all those theories in depth is beyond the scope of this book. Besides, what's going to be most useful to you is a good dose of common sense and pragmatism. There's no point quoting scientific theories while stuffing in those last few mouthfuls of cake 'because it's a shame to waste it'. And you don't need theorems to know when you've eaten to excess!

Satiety signals can differ slightly from person to person, so as well as being mindful of your eating you also need to learn how to interpret what you are feeling so that you can pinpoint your own individual fullness threshold. It's a form of self-awareness, listening to your body and your mind to understand what the sensations are for you, a bit like knowing how much you can drink before you become drunk! In my case, if I feel a tightness and/or pressure just below my solar plexus and across the top of my abdomen, as well as a sort of fatigue, then I've already eaten too much. Eating any more suddenly feels like more of an effort than a pleasure, and I feel weighed down by each extra mouthful. The trick is to find and acknowledge your own fullness feelings and then act on them day after day until the process of stopping eating when you are full becomes an ingrained habit.

But what if you are distracted from this important self-awareness? If you're eating while doing other things, like watching TV, walking, talking a lot, feeling rushed or stressed, or being in a stimulating environment, will you will have the focus to recognize your sensations of fullness before you 'tip the balance' and overeat?

And if there's a bunch of other things going on during your meal, will you be eating with enough attention to the tastes, textures and aromas which are a key part of feeling psychologically satisfied and nurtured?

Having distractions present while you are eating will also leave you less satisfied by your food and perhaps even encourage you to eat faster, therefore consume more calories in less time. Can you imagine why McDonald's and other fast-food providers might use music, crowded eating areas, bright lights, music and other distractions in their restaurants?

What's the conclusion?

Ditch the distractions and be totally committed to the taste, texture, feel and experience that make food that much *more* than just something to fill us up!

Now take a piece of paper and take ten minutes to write down 25 things that might distract you from concentrating on your food. Be honest and open and let your pen do the talking. Push yourself – 25 isn't that many at all (you've surely been distracted from your food more than 25 times in your life?)

Now take five minutes to review what you've written and draw conclusions, as follows:

1. 'What steps am I going to take from now on to prevent being distracted from concentrating on mindful eating?

2. 'What changes am I going to make to my mealtimes (where and when I eat, who I eat with?)'

3. 'What are my strategies going to be from now on to ensure that I'm enjoying an uninterrupted, complete experience of nurturing myself with healthy food and eating mindfully?'

Write down your strategies.

Now sign a commitment to yourself to follow these strategies from now on:

> 'From now on I am committed to ditching the distractions so that I can commit to eating mindfully and recognizing when I am full. I am committing to following these strategies to empower myself to do this.'

Being distracted from what you are eating is not a recipe for enjoying your food *or* for losing or controlling weight. So, ditch the TV, ignore the telephone, think twice about strolling along eating that ice-cream in summer and certainly quit tapping on your laptop with your packed lunch beside you!

Key Points to Remember
- The *most important* weapon in the fight against overeating is the ability to recognize when you are full – which is difficult to gauge if your brain is occupied elsewhere!
- Having distractions present while you are eating you will also leave you less satisfied by your food and perhaps even encourage you to eat faster, consuming more calories in less time.
- So *ditch the distractions* and be totally committed to the taste, texture, feel and experience that make food that much *more* than just something to fill us up!

Key Number Twenty-Two

Take a Moment, Count to Ten

The old advice to count to ten has a lot going for it! My mentor Steve Linder says, 'Putting emotion before reason is dangerous both in business and in life.' Steve knows a thing or two about the balance between emotion and reason, having spent years studying stock market psychology. At 24 he sold his online stock-trading company to E-Trade for $14m and reached the top of corporate America as CIO of Bank of America. After 9/11, he quit to empower people to live their potential. As the founder of the most advanced NLP training company in the world today, he has the opportunity to observe the balance between reason and emotion daily!

The multi-millionaire educator Robert Kiyosaki advocates the power of stopping and analysing really concisely in his famous book *Rich Dad, Poor Dad*:

> 'Stop what you are doing. In other words, take a break and assess what is working and what is not working. The definition of insanity is doing the same thing and expecting a different result. Stop doing what is not working and look for something new to do.'[37]

Many unwise decisions are made as a result of instinctive actions and 'knee-jerk' reactions – basically, when emotion trumps reason. We've all done it – and we've all regretted it afterwards. So, remember what your mother used to tell you: 'Stop and count to ten!'

Can you think of ten examples where this advice would have served you well?

Now take pen and paper and write them down...

It's the power of a simple ten seconds. Remember, every great decision ever made was made in ten seconds or fewer! Ten seconds can change your life. You can decide to throw the gun down, shut the fridge door, turn down that adulterous rendezvous that would ruin your marriage, pour the whiskey down the sink, all in ten seconds!

Ten seconds to decide to make your life better. Ten seconds to serve yourself. Ten seconds to serve others. Ten seconds to serve yourself *and* others! Wow! How powerful are ten seconds when you use them to think wisely?

Ask yourself:

> 'Can I spare ten seconds of a lifetime to make the right decision?'

> 'Will I change my world by sparing ten seconds to make the right decisions again and again?'

You really *can* change your world in an instant: when you know what you want in life. If you already know what you want, the groundwork is laid and you just have to follow through with making sure your decisions match what you desire!

Steve Linder calls matching your decisions with your goals *congruency* – basically, it's lining up your actions with your aims.

Ask yourself:

> 'When am I going to start lining up my actions with my aims?'

This is something I know all about. Whenever I get the urge to eat chocolate biscuits or French fries or forego my daily 20-minute jog, I take ten seconds to remind myself of my *identity* and my *mission in life*. I say to myself, 'I'm the author of a bestselling book, I'm a "self-optimizer" and I'm an expert in helping people to achieve their aims in life! Do French fries or chocolate biscuits or sitting on the couch fit into my identity? Will they help me achieve my aims in life?'

Of course the answer is a resounding 'No!' And in those ten seconds I have realized it.

When you create goals for yourself, you are also creating a new *identity* for yourself: as someone who will do what it takes to reach those goals. For example, just as some people put pictures on the fridge of a slimmer self, I have pictures in my mind of how I see my ideal identity – which I'm moving closer to every day of my life. And these pictures don't include me eating chocolate biscuits or French fries or compromising on exercising daily.

Creating this new identity means being self-aware, not acting compulsively and thinking through actions all the way to their outcome! It means standing back and taking ten seconds to ask yourself questions like:

- 'Do I feel like eating without being hungry? Is that good? Does it serve me and my goal?'
- 'Do I want to keep on eating when actually I'm already full? Is that wise? Does it serve me and my goal?'
- 'Do I feel like snacking for emotional reasons? Is that going to make me feel better in the long run or worse? Does it serve me and my goal?'

That small pause to clarify things helps to *break the pattern of habits that don't serve you.*

It can also work when the course of action is not quite so clear-cut, for example when you're tossing up whether to go out jogging in the rain or to lie curled up in bed. You take a small pause and think over the *consequences* (outcome) of your decision:

- 'How will this decision affect me *now*?'
- 'How will this decision affect my long-term goals?'

To take another example, I jog to increase my fitness levels, but I only do 15–25 minutes a day. Because this isn't a huge amount of time, every day adds up, so not jogging (however comfortable that decision might seem when I'm lying in bed!) will jeopardize my ongoing exercise routine for the week and make me feel sluggish. When I'm fit and well, the benefits of jogging for 20 minutes (with a waterproof jacket on if it's raining!) actually far outweigh 20 minutes of lying cosily and lazily in bed. Decision made!

On the other hand, if I had a sore throat one day, I might decide it was a better strategy to not push my immune system to the limit and risk coming down with a cold, as I'd be jeopardizing my exercise routine for the whole week! In this case I'd be thinking more of my long-term goals.

Here are some other things to be aware of:

1. Be clear about your goal, so your decisions can be made quickly.
2. Go with what you *know* you should do, not what you *want* to do.
3. Be aware of what's on the line and what's at stake!
4. Realize that counting to ten is all about interrupting an old behaviour pattern and inserting a *new* one instead. You're basically changing strategies!
5. When you rush ahead doing what you've always done, there's no time to make a different choice. Counting to ten gives you the gift of a moment to decide to act differently. Will you accept that gift and honour the opportunity?

In his brilliant book *The End of Overeating*, Dr David Kessler talks about what he calls 'effective intervention'. He describes this as 'the knowledge that we have a moment of choice – *but only a moment* – to recognize what is about to happen and do something else instead'.[38] That's the moment when we can stop and count to ten!

Then, says Dr Kessler, 'we can practice new behaviours and learn new thoughts to keep the old ones at bay. Eventually these become as automatic as our past responses, and when they do, the [old] stimulus begins to cool.'[39]

Dr Kessler also quotes Matthew State, professor of child psychiatry and genetics at Yale School of Medicine, who says that: 'You have to ask people to specifically pay attention so that they can … self-monitor. Once they pay attention, they have a capacity to extinguish the [unwanted] behaviour.'[40]

How about an example? Say you find yourself at a lunch or dinner buffet. (By the way, isn't it strange that buffets are designed so you can come back for more, but on the first serving people pile their plates so high you'd think food was about to be rationed forever?)

Do you:

a) Rush ahead, join the queue and pile your plate high with everything – the old 'your eye is bigger than your stomach' scenario?

b) Stop for a moment, count to ten and decide to choose healthier options, be more restrained and, if you want to pile your plate up, pile it up with veggies and salad instead?

OK, here's another strategy you can follow when you feel you are about to make a decision that doesn't serve you positively. It's easy to remember because it's based on what you learned as a child when your mum was teaching you to cross the road safely: '*Stop, look and listen.*'

Say you are just going to open the biscuit tin and eat a biscuit, but you're not really hungry, are you?

1. *Stop.* (*Before* you put that biscuit into your mouth!)
2. *Look* at the situation. ('I was just about to greedily stuff this biscuit into my mouth and I'm not even hungry!')
3. *Listen* to your internal dialogue, what your thoughts are saying to you. Ask the part of you that wants to rush in like a fool what it wants. For example: 'Part of me says I'm hungry. Why does it want the biscuit? It wants it because it tastes good, and that makes me feel good.')

And now you use it in reverse: '*Listen, look, go!*'

1. *Listen* to your heart, the part of you that wants to serve your best interests. ('I know you want to feel good, but compulsive eating when you aren't hungry isn't going to make you happy! You might enjoy the biscuit while it's in your mouth, but how are you going to feel afterwards?')
2. *Look* for a replacement strategy. ('Instead of eating this biscuit, I'm going to put it back in the tin, close the lid and feel good about making the right choice. I'm going to exit the kitchen right now and call a friend instead – which will make me feel happy.')
3. *Go* ahead with taking positive action. Then congratulate yourself on your great decision and ask yourself, 'What have I learned? How can I use this again? How can I share this?'

Let's take an example of this strategy in action. Jane has just had a stressful day at work and is walking past a doughnut shop on the way back to her car. She smells that sticky, sweet smell wafting out of the shop and feels the urge to go in and buy a box of doughnuts. She feels she just can't resist that melting, buttery dough. But she also knows she always feels very guilty after she's licked every last smear of caramel frosting off her fingers, especially since she's already overweight and doughnuts never fill her up, just make her feel hungrier and all the more out of control.

Normally she'd walk into the shop as soon as she has the urge, but today she:

1. *Stops* on the street.
2. *Looks* at the situation with detachment, telling herself, 'In this moment I have a choice whether to walk into that shop and buy a box of doughnuts or cross the road and walk away.'
3. Now she *listens* to her internal dialogue, to the part of her that wants the doughnuts: 'I've had a hard day at work and I'm tired. I need something to give me a boost and cheer me up. Doughnuts are sweet and I'll feel great while I'm eating them.'

Then she reverses the process. She:

1. *Listens* to her heart, the part of her that wants to serve her positively: 'If I walk into that shop now, how will I feel when I've eaten those caramel frosted doughnuts? Last time I didn't feel energized and cheered up, I just felt disgusted and guilty, and the doughnuts were really quite sickly, after all! And that's several hundred calories I don't want on my hips, which will blow the healthy food I've eaten today out of the water. Eating doughnuts won't cheer me up or make me feel energized at all!'
2. She *looks* for a replacement strategy: 'How about walking past the shop and getting to the car quickly instead so I can drive home? I can put on some nice music when I'm home and relax, have a soothing shower, then fix myself a light dinner! And I'll feel so good about meeting my needs in a way that won't make me fat and guilty but will nurture me instead!'
3. Now Jane says, '*Go!*' and walks past the shop, back to her car. As soon as she turns the corner, the stimulus and craving subside. It's over! She unlocks her car, gets in and sits back against the seat with a sigh of relief. It was easy, after all! And instead of following her old behaviour, she's just wired a new strategy into her brain!

When she gets back home, she congratulates herself on her great decision and tells herself, 'I've learned that when I'm tired and fed up I don't have to rely on having sugary snacks to give me a boost. I can find healthier ways to satisfy that need for energy and pleasure. I'm going to remember this next time I feel tired or low. If I can do it once, I can do it again! And I'm going to tell all my friends I've quit eating doughnuts!'

Note that Jane is *not* using willpower. There is no clash of desire against discipline. She is still fulfilling the need to do something to relieve her tiredness and cheer herself up, but she's fulfilling it in a positive way.

Habit helps. As we learned way back at beginning of this book, when we repeat an action it is 'hard-wired' into our brain, but by replacing it with a different action, we can rewire the brain. Then the *stimulus* might still be there, but the *response* will be different.

The Three Power Questions

Here are the three great questions Jane asks herself when she's made that change in behaviour, or 'rewired her strategy', to put it in Neurostrategy terms:

1. 'What have I learned?'
2. 'How can I use this again?'
3. 'How can I share this?'

You can ask yourself these questions too!

Key Points to Remember

- When you're not sure about a course of action or you want to make sure you're making decisions which fit in with your goals, just take a moment, count to ten and give yourself the space to stop and think.
- Stopping and counting to ten can also work when the course of action is not clear-cut.
- Use the moment's pause to reconnect with your goals. Ask yourself what you *really* want so you can align your actions with your aim.
- Use the strategy *Stop, look and listen* to understand your urges and evaluate your feelings so you have the power to prevent self-sabotage, then use *Listen, look, go!* to tune into taking positive action that will serve you best.
- You don't need willpower, just a change in strategy, and it can be effortless!
- Afterwards, ask yourself, *'What have I learned? How can I use this again? How can I share this?'*

Key Number Twenty-Three

Thirsty?

When we're dehydrated, we feel a physical need crying to be filled up. This isn't surprising, when we consider how important H20 is to us: water comprises up to 60 per cent of our body, 70 per cent of our brain, 90 per cent of our lungs, 22 per cent of our bones and over 80 per cent of our blood![41] We have to replace almost two and a half litres of water per day through drinks and the food we ingest. The carbohydrates and proteins which fuel us are metabolized and transported through the bloodstream by water. Waste material is also transported out of the body (water being an essential dissolving agent).

According to the US Geological Survey's Water Science for Schools website, babies have the largest percentage of body water, about 78 per cent at birth, dropping to about 65 per cent at one year of age. Adult men have about 60 per cent, adult women about 55 per cent.[42] Because fat tissue contains less water than lean tissue, people with more fat have less body water as a percentage than those who are leaner.

When you drink a large glass of water you'll often find that the physical need to fill up was just that – like a car at a petrol pump, it was fluid that was needed, not food! However, so many people just interpret that 'empty' signal as hunger for food, and eat. What do you think is the result of this happening again and again?

The old advice that you'll lose weight if you drink a glass of water before a meal maybe wasn't about filling up the stomach with water at all – water *won't* fill up your stomach for any length of time, especially an empty stomach: you'll just visit the bathroom more! – but about not confusing hunger with thirst.

Try drinking a large glass of refreshing water every time you feel the urge to eat and you'll be surprised how often the desire for food disappears. Keep a large brightly coloured cup and jug of freshly filtered water close at hand, in the centre of your kitchen counter, and a bottle of mineral water on your desk at work. Flavouring water with a slice of apple, orange, lemon or lime (or a sprig of fresh mint) is also a wonderful treat – which I thoroughly enjoyed at a spa recently!

The more you drink water regularly to quench your thirst and prevent dehydration, the more you'll be able to recognize the difference between hunger and thirst. Real hunger is quite unmistakeable: your tummy will be grumbling, legs feeling weak and so on.

The desire to eat lots of water-rich fruit can be another sign of dehydration. If your body needs the water in the fruit, it's better to drink the water you need from a glass, because you'd have to eat an awful lot of fruit to satisfy the thirst craving! Fruit is a healthier snack than cakes and biscuits, but don't forget that most fruit is high in sugars and anyone planning to lose excess weight should exercise caution and prioritize low-GI fruit (check out *'Powerful Food Habit number 4'* in Chapter 4) such as berries, forest fruits and green apples; those suffering from irritable bowel syndrome should also note that fructose (fruit sugar) can be a trigger. (For more information on fructose, see *Chapter 5*, which explains about *'High-Fructose Corn Syrup'* and *'The Sugar Trap'.*)

In any event, it is wise to start a meal with a glass of water. You'll feel calmer and more balanced when you're fully hydrated – and you'll eat more mindfully as a result!

Whatever you do, ignore the old myth about not drinking with a meal. That was more to do with too many fizzy drinks or alcohol interfering with digestion, or possibly with the fact that many juices and drinks are high in sugar and calories. If you consume high-calorie drinks you'll have to take their caloric value into consideration, but combining them with a meal (or not) won't have any effect on the energy they provide! Remember that fizzy drinks are packed full of added sugar, and the carbonated bubbles can cause indigestion and bloating. If you want to lose weight and keep it off, laying off the fizzy drinks is a wise move – including 'diet' coke and artificially-sweetened drinks which may enhance sugar cravings (instead of the other way round) and may actually cause you to put on weight![43]

Carbonated mineral water is fine in moderation, but do take note of the sodium (salt) content – some fancy mineral waters can be quite high in sodium, which encourages water retention and bloating. For the same reason children shouldn't be given mineral water to drink. Filtered (and even better, distilled or purified) water is preferable to tap water, and much safer for your health. Tap water can contain trace elements of various unhealthy substances – whether within legal levels or not, it's best to avoid them altogether (I myself have suffered higher than safe levels of lead in my body due to lead water pipes in the houses I've lived in).

Hot drinks, on the other hand, can be diuretic, which means that they encourage the body to release water through the urine – which takes you back to being dehydrated! Dr Isaac Jones suggests drinking at least one cup of water to one cup of coffee or tea to make up for the diuretic effect of the hot drink. Caffeinated coffee and non-herbal teas also contain caffeine and tannin, mild stimulants which enhance further the diuretic effect – in excess, encouraging mild dehydration. It is advisable to limit these, or you'll find yourself taking frequent trips to the bathroom.

There are many diets which advocate losing weight through increasing coffee or tea intake. Realistically, it's the diuretic effect of these drinks which provides an artificial sense of weight loss (it's nothing more than water loss), as well as the temporary sensation of filling up the stomach (with liquid). Neither of these will cause actual weight loss or burn fat to any notable extent.[44]

Important Note

Note that there is such thing as drinking *too much* water. People with some heart conditions, high blood pressure, swelling of the lower legs (oedema) and kidney problems should avoid excessive water consumption. Please consult your doctor for detailed advice.

Too much water can also disrupt digestion by diluting stomach acid. In extreme cases – 'water intoxication' – it can even prove fatal. Water intoxication occurs when the electrolytes in the body are so diluted that they are unable to maintain cellular water balance. A couple of large glasses of water are the most that should be drunk at any one sitting. As we are learning, *moderation*, not excess, is the key to healthy eating and drinking!

Please also note that due to the chemicals which leach out of plastic bottles, especially when exposed to sunlight, it is advisable to store water in glass rather than plastic (aluminium cans can also leach particles).

Key Points to Remember
- If you feel a need to fill yourself up, first try a large glass of water – your body could be quite simply thirsty instead of hungry. Thirst being mistaken for hunger is a common cause of overeating.
- In any event, it is wise to start a meal with a glass of water. You'll feel more balanced and calm when you're fully hydrated – and you'll eat more mindfully as a result.
- If you want to lose weight, laying off the fizzy drinks is a wise move – including 'diet' coke and artificially sweetened drinks.

- Excessive consumption of hot drinks has a diuretic effect and may actually lead to dehydration. Drinking hot drinks will not cause weight loss alone.
- Make sure you drink enough water, but don't drink it to excess. Moderation is the key.

Key Number Twenty-Four

Why Do You Eat When You're Not Hungry?

Food is bundled up with a whole universe of associations, having nurtured us from birth onwards, from mother's milk to childhood treats, from hot chocolate in winter to ice-cream in summer. All around the world, even in the poorest countries, food means so much more than simple nutrition. It is offered as a symbol of celebration, religion, culture, unity, even fertility. There is food to fit any occasion, enhance any mood. It is a sign of hospitality, of greeting, of negotiation, of peace – there's nothing more important than food!

It's great to bring people together and celebrate and share that most basic of needs, eating! But we mustn't forget that food's primary function is to provide nutrition. If we do forget that, is it any surprise that we get overweight? And if we use food as an emotional prop, or a sticking plaster to cover our woes, we aren't respecting it at all, we're abusing it. Food is sacred for its ability to heal and nurture. It shouldn't be a drug.

However, modern man is increasingly creating food that has lost touch with its nutritional purpose and instead is crammed full of empty calories, artificial additives, fat, sugar and salt. We all know what 'junk' food is – some of us even eat it! But did you know that even *non*-fast-food restaurants are becoming very clever at producing food that's loaded and layered with fat, sugar and salt? Dr. David Kessler, author of *The End of Overeating*, describes the 'Shanghai Lobster with spicy ginger curry sauce and crispy spinach' at Chinois, Wolfgang Puck's renowned restaurant in Santa Monica. The lobster was fried in peanut oil then baked in the oven and 'when it arrived ... nothing about its appearance revealed the amount of fat it contained'. [45]

Plenty of 'savoury' foods nowadays contain copious amounts of sugar, especially those with sauces, smoke or barbecue flavourings, dressings, and so on – even the innocent-sounding soup is definitely not immune to being sugar-loaded. 'Hedonic' food like this, laced with fat, salt and sugar, produces a chemical reaction in the body which can be as addictive as a drug. It provides instant gratification but not long-term nurturing – not very different from any other sort of drug, in fact.[46]

The modern obesity epidemic is linked to two main factors:

1. Consumption of these dangerously 'engineered' modern foods (which David Kessler calls 'hyperpalatable').
2. Exaggerated overeating, compulsive eating, eating for comfort...

Sadly, food is often used to fill a void which is psychological and not physical, an emotional 'hole' which is instinctively crying out to be filled and is mistaken for that emptiness when a stomach cries out in hunger.

In *Think Thin, Be Thin,* Doris Wild Helmering and Dianne Hales offer up these rules to understand whether your hunger is physical or emotional:

- *Physical Hunger* builds gradually; strikes below the neck (e.g. a growling stomach); occurs several hours after a meal; goes away when full; eating leads to a feeling of satisfaction.
- *Emotional Hunger* develops suddenly; strikes above the neck (e.g. a 'taste' for ice cream); is unrelated to time; persists despite fullness; eating leads to guilt and shame.[47]

If we've been given food to cheer us up since birth, is it little wonder that we confuse emotional emptiness with physical hunger? The worst aspect is that emotional eating's a totally self-defeating pattern – you're not removing the difficult emotions by eating over them, merely adding to them by becoming fat and miserable!

Here are some common emotions which cause people to reach for comfort in the form of food:

- loneliness
- sadness
- despair
- boredom
- frustration
- anger
- fear
- guilt
- hurt
- anxiety
- impatience/anticipation
- excitement
- low self-esteem
- feeling out of control

And if you are prone to emotional eating, here's a really powerful exercise:

Go through the list of 14 emotions above and think of *specific* situations when you've stuffed food into your mouth while feeling overwhelmed (or underwhelmed!) by these emotions.

Now, take a pen and a piece of paper and write down, in the form of headings, the 14 emotions listed above. Leave lots of space beneath them. You can even use a separate sheet for each.

Under each heading, write down a time you've overeaten (or would commonly overeat) when feeling the emotion. Put in as much detail as possible. Please also catalogue the various foods you'd feel like eating (or have eaten) under these circumstances.

If you can't think of a specific occasion, generalize according to when you know you *might or would* feel tempted to eat while feeling this emotion.

Take especial note of any feelings of shame and guilt which pop up. Shame and guilt indicate valuable learning opportunities for change! So, don't ignore them, try to hide from them or push them away. Think of them like the flags at the holes on a golf course – they're there to tell you where to *aim* so you can really improve your life!

Now, for each example, ask yourself:

- Did you feel better or worse by eating in response to emotion?
- Did eating in response to emotion help to remove any issues or problems or uncomfortable emotions?
- Did eating in response to emotion make a long-term contribution to solving the problem or relieving your state of mind?
- Did eating in response to emotion serve to aggravate your misery (making you feel fat, sick, full, miserable, worse, out of control)?

You can put ticks or crosses by each example, if it helps.

Now for each of the 14 examples, complete these sentences:

- 'This disgusts me because...'
- 'Eating [the food] will never make things better in this case because...'

Again, go into as much detail as possible.

You are now going to pen your own commitment to stopping emotional eating:

> 'I commit, from this moment on, to eating only when I'm hungry and balanced. If I ever feel [emotion], instead of eating [food], I commit to [your new strategy, for example calling a friend and arranging something fun]! Whenever I feel [emotion], I will not disgust myself by eating food I do not need. Instead, I am committed to taking positive action by [strategy] so that I will not only feel better but also lose weight!'

I know that there's a lot of writing going on here! But believe me, the best way to consolidate our aims is to write them down. I speak to a lot of very successful people and renowned entrepreneurs, and I haven't yet met one who doesn't write down their goals and commitments on a regular basis.

Now, let's talk about overeating at happy times – festive times of celebration, weddings, parties or a meal out with loved ones. There are all sorts of 'treats' represented by food, from a cake and hot chocolate with a girlfriend in winter to a cocktail by the pool in summer – that one gives me a nice breezy feeling just thinking of it! These are also times when we may overeat due to emotion, but in this case the emotions are positive ones. The point, however, is that it's still overeating...

In a nutshell, please don't spoil great times by overeating. Just enjoy your food in moderation according to what's good for you!

Here's a mantra you can repeat if you wish:

'Respect the food that nurtures you! Respect your appetite and respect yourself!'

Of course in some situations, as mentioned earlier, the pride of the cook, the desire for acknowledgement and various social dynamics may be involved. Remember 'food pushers'? Such situations need to be left to your own judgement, but *remember that overeating is habit-forming*. If you overeat to be polite – or for any other reason – you do so at your own peril.

There is nothing wrong with celebrating the wonderful and amazing universe of food. It is one of life's great pleasures. And we can all be forgiven for overindulging a little during festive occasions, as long we can put it into perspective, and put moderation back on the menu the very next day. But ask yourself, 'What is a healthy relationship with food?'

Here's your answer: 'It's knowing the difference between choice and compulsion and being able to make that choice and weigh up the pros and cons. It's actually a healthy relationship with yourself!'

Important Note

If you cannot have a healthy relationship with food and consistently overeat for emotional reasons, are unable to address this on your own and believe you may have an eating disorder, then please do seek help from a qualified professional. Do not underestimate the fact that eating disorders are highly addictive and dangerous, and can even be life-threatening at their most extreme. This book is not intended to dispense or replace the advice of a qualified medical practitioner.

Key Points to Remember
- Food is often used as a prop, comforter or sticking plaster. If you suspect you are using food in this way (emotional or compulsive eating) then please take a long, hard look at your behaviour and find an alternative, healthy solution to your immediate need (for comfort or otherwise).
- If there is a consistent and constant exaggeration and indulgence, there may well be a lifestyle change to consider, or an emotional reason for excess to be confronted.
- Food is also a key element in celebrations, but do beware of overdoing it and make sure you balance out any excesses.
- Be sensitive when there is a host who has an emotional attachment to their role as provider of food.
- It's knowing the difference between choosing rationally and enjoying what you eat and compulsively reaching for food which you don't require that denotes a healthy relationship with food – and with yourself.

Key Number Twenty-Five

Delay your Gratification...

Whenever I think of the concept of 'delayed gratification', which we touched on briefly earlier, I think of Duncan Bannatyne. Duncan's the Scottish entrepreneur well-known in the UK as a judge on the BBC TV show *Dragon's Den*, evaluating the pitches of aspiring entrepreneurs. He also has a chain of fitness clubs throughout the British Isles. His is a real rags-to-riches tale which anyone can learn from.

In 2010, according to *The Sunday Times* rich list, Duncan Bannatyne's net worth was £320 million, but just over 30 years before that he was sitting almost penniless on a beach on the island of Jersey with no career, no formal education and a criminal record! But an article about the millionaire Alan Sugar (now Lord Sugar) in the newspaper he had read over breakfast made him sit up and take note. He vowed to become a millionaire and give his future children what he'd never had.

Duncan's rise to riches depended on one thing: delayed gratification. Never one for an extravagant lifestyle while he was building his fortune, he carefully invested his earnings with the next goal and business venture in mind. He didn't blow his cash on expensive houses and a lavish lifestyle until he had plenty to spare! In his autobiography, he talks of the period leading up to his first big gamble (a residential care home business, which would later net him millions). At one point he put everything he owned into the venture, selling not only the roof over his head but his stereo, car and, actually, any possession of any value – much to his wife's horror! He sacrificed almost everything in the short term in order to push through a deal which would reap him a greater reward in the longer term. He risked a lot, but the reward was even greater!

This is exactly what 'delayed gratification' means: making sacrifices in the present in order to reach a valuable goal in the future. The concept is valid for any area of life. In my case, if I hadn't put in four hours of writing almost every day, sacrificing hobbies, socializing, relaxation and part of my holidays too, you wouldn't be reading this book! Another example: when I was at college I never spent money at the bar or café, or on clothes or movies or alcohol: I saved it towards a second-hand car and a mobile phone (the size of a brick!) and I was the envy of many of my fellow students. I used to charge people to use my phone. I also got a good job at Hewlett-Packard in my gap year because I had that car. The payback for missing out on paying for rounds of drinks at the bar was great!

Similarly, anyone who wants to be successful at sports knows that it's necessary to put in daily workouts and training sessions. As gruelling as they may be while muscles are burning, there's a goal propelling the athlete or rower or ballet dancer through the pain barrier!

And if you want to be slim and at your most attractive, certainly there is work to be done: work on not overeating, on making the right nutritional choices, on building physical exercise into your routine, on staying calm and balanced and eating slowly, to mention just a few. There is no gain without effort, so get real. There are no shortcuts. 'You get out what you put in,' says a friend of mine who plays competitive tennis (thanks, James). That's really true both in sport and in life!

When you understand that a little hard work or initial discomfort in the present can lead to great rewards in the future, you open the door to the success waiting just round the corner!

The good news is that to be relatively fit and pleasingly slim, you don't need starvation diets or gruelling exercise, just constant attention and a few changes in habit and lifestyle – pleasant and happy changes!

To keep your motivation high, you need to consolidate your vision of what you're aiming at. This is where visualization comes in. Remember that because the unconscious mind doesn't differentiate between reality and vivid imagination, and it harnesses all our resources toward producing what we visualize. That's why we are what we imagine ourselves to be!

Just remember that in the Bank of Delayed Gratification, there are *no* payment holidays, so keep your goal in mind and make your effort consistent. You have to keep on making payments to get the balance you aim for!

Now let's talk a bit more about the opposite of delayed gratification – instant gratification. It seems that our society is becoming more and more about that instant hit: fast fame, fast money, fast cars, fast sex – not forgetting fast food!

My English grandmother used to say, 'A little bit of what you fancy does you good.' She was an eternally slim lady of regal elegance – who also enjoyed helping herself to her favourite box of chocolates every day after dinner! Needless to say, she was measured in everything she did. And her Jaeger suits always fit her immaculately!

In fact, being able to compensate from day to day and week to week is a natural process which our ancestors were used to, depending on whether food was plentiful or less so, and this process is known as *homoeostasis*. It's basically the ability to self-regulate and turn too much or too little into a balance overall. When my grandmother ate chocolate, she naturally ate less of other foods. But things have changed in recent years.

Dr David Kessler, author of *The End of Overeating*, argues that we're losing this ability to self-regulate. He and other enlightened physicians now believe that the availability of highly stimulating fast foods is tapping into our brain's reward system and overriding homoeostatis.[48] The brain is becoming wired in the wrong way: people are looking to fat, salt, sugar and calorie-laden, nutrition-empty foods to provide instant reward through taste alone.[49] No delayed gratification there then!

Neuroscientist Edmund Rolls, from a team at Oxford University, found out that part of the brain actually calculates when you should '*stop* partaking in something pleasurable',[50] i.e. when a reward loses its appeal, when it just doesn't do it for you anymore (technically that's known as 'sensory-specific satiety').

Now if an immediate reward can lose its appeal that easily, then we are really not 'slaves to instant gratification'[51] after all. It appears that we can actually gain pleasure from *delaying our pleasure*. In fact, Rolls also found that the abstract concept of future financial reward could produce changes in brain activity. It seems that the chance of a future reward can be as powerful – if not more so – than immediate reward![52]

When I first learned this, I tested it on my own kids! Both of them – five and six years old at the time – chose the chance to have two chocolate treats the following day instead of one immediately. And these are children who only have 'chocolate day' once a week! Even for them, the promise of a greater delayed reward was perceived as more valuable than an immediate one. Even if they had to wait a whole day – very long as far as a five-year-old child and chocolate is concerned!

Now please take pen and paper and write this down:

> '*The chance of a future reward is more powerful than immediate reward.*'

Now take a few moments and jot down some examples from your own life, either of times when this has come true for you, or of future rewards you have in mind.

Now write down what you're going to do in the present to increase the chance of that future reward. Take 10–15 minutes to do this exercise, because it's a powerful one.

When you translate this to losing weight, you have two scenarios:
- Eat the doughnut now and get that sugar hit and great taste for a few seconds.
- Forego the doughnut and feel more empowered, healthier and on the way to getting fitter and slimmer!

Thinking of the long-term benefit really can be much more powerful than simply giving into temptation and 'living for the moment'. Focusing on the long-term benefit changes short-term effort into a feeling of pleasure, anticipation … and pride!

When we ignore a stimulus or craving that wouldn't have served us, often our pride at acting positively isn't immediately obvious. After all, we're busy going through effort (even pain!) to make the right decision, which isn't always easy in the moment. But when you reconnect with the pride and joy you get from serving yourself positively, these very feelings can become your *immediate reward*, and guess what?! – they're not even fattening!

In this way, there's no sacrifice. What's more, you're on the path to reaping even greater rewards later on. That's because every time you respect yourself and make a decision that will make you healthier in the present moment, you are also taking great strides forward along the path to health and self-esteem in the future.

When I jog every day, it's not always easy. Sometimes my muscles burn and I feel really tired. But I get such pleasure from visualizing how toned and fit I'm becoming – I do this as I run! – that the exertion doesn't even count in the equation!

And you know what? The gratification isn't delayed for long. Before you know it you'll be reaping the rewards!

Key Points to Remember
- Delayed gratification means making sacrifices in the present in order to reach a valuable goal in the future.
- Help yourself by visualizing the goals you are aiming for.
- It has been proven that the chance of a future reward is more powerful than immediate reward.
- Ultimately, it's not a sacrifice because the pride and joy you get from serving yourself positively become your immediate reward. And you're on the path to reaping even greater rewards later on.

Key Number Twenty-Six

Don't Worry, Be Happy!

Let me introduce you to something called 'positive psychology'. Sounds good, doesn't it? It began in 1998 when Martin Seligman, its founding father, pointed out that clinical psychology had until then concentrated on overcoming problems and mental illness: a really negative focus. In contrast, positive psychology focuses on how to improve thinking abilities and perception. It is being used increasingly by coaches, counsellors and other professionals to help people just like you expand and enrich their lives, develop their skills, enjoy success and gain real results!

In a nutshell, the key factor of positive psychology is optimism. So anyone can apply it to their life! An optimistic frame of mind can help anyone to achieve more, whether their goal is to lose weight, increase self-confidence, enhance critical thinking and open-mindedness, or even improve the way they deal with stress – lab and survey research has indicated that positive emotions have positive effects on the cardiovascular system, decreasing heart rate, lowering blood sugar, and so on![53]

Here are a few simple steps you can take effortlessly and straight away:

Focus on What You Can Do *Now*

If we spend our time regretting the past (which is gone) and worrying about the future (which is yet to come), we are focusing on what doesn't exist! Because, in actual fact, all we have is the present. It doesn't matter what you did in the past, and tomorrow doesn't exist either – it's just an extension of today. *Today* is the day you can create a new healthy habit or make improvements to yourself and your world: today, day after day after day!

It is only by concentrating on the present that we can make amends for our past and create our future. With weight loss, as in everything else, it's what we do *now* that counts: what we eat *now*, the exercise we take *now* and the thoughts we have *now*.

By taking positive and targeted action, and concentrating on our experience of the here and now, we take control of our lives: we stop dwelling on unhappiness from the past and fear of the future. We discover that our everyday experiences are ready to be enjoyed!

Savour the Present

Enjoy the positive feelings that are part of your everyday life: your interests, hobbies, loved ones, fun experiences, etc. Positive psychology talks about a 'life of engagement'. When you *engage with what you are engaged in*, you increase in confidence and happiness because you experience life more closely and more deeply.

When you immerse yourself in what you're currently doing, how you feel and where you are, you're being mindful. You are also filling and engaging your mind and senses, so you don't need artificial stimulation or distractions to make you feel good. When you savour the pleasures of the moment, you'll be more satisfied. This is, of course, not only useful in weight loss but also in creating a greater sense of satisfaction in general!

Serve Others and Add Value

We derive well-being and meaning from being part of something greater than ourselves. So, how about joining a social group, contributing in some way to your local community, doing a favour for a friend or volunteering in some way? How about enhancing the relationships you have with your family and relatives and making some extra-special gesture or gestures they'll never forget? How about seeing where you can add extra value at work to your bosses, colleagues or clients – you'll be surprised how much it's appreciated when they realize you don't actually want anything in exchange!

When you add value to others, rewards flow back to you in the form of optimism, support, joy and confidence – and very often success too.

Adding value to others can be as simple as joining a club where you are all helping each other to achieve your goals. If you find it hard to get fit, for example, why not join a fitness class, or a local support group, or get sponsorship for a walk in aid of a charity close to your heart – this will give you impetus to succeed and plenty of sponsors cheering you on! One of the reasons why the Weight Watchers slimming programme has been so successful is because of the sense of community its participants feel.

Serving others also means *quitting being selfish* where being selfish serves no one, including yourself. Many people decide to lose weight, for example, when they realize their relationship with their children is compromised. Perhaps they are unable to run around, play sport or have enough energy for their kids. They suddenly realize that their actions affect other people, not just themselves, and that to continue down the same route won't just rob themselves of opportunity, but rob their kids of opportunity too – the opportunity to have parents who are healthy and fit and able to share in the joys of life!

Serving others may mean turning to religion or spirituality for comfort. Anything which is greater than the individual and extends out to encompass others can give us a positive sense of belonging, meaning and purpose, and empower us to achieve our goals and make improvements in our lives.

Serving others also takes the focus off 'me, me me' … or 'you, you, you'. A little objectivity is a good thing, helping us to see ourselves as others see us. It may be a shock – but one that shocks us into positive action! Your best friend, your spouse and your mother, for example, are people who can be honest with you about where you can improve your giving. But why wait for them to tell you when we all know deep down where we're being selfish? Listen to your instincts and act on them to improve your relationships!

When you are happy and contributing to the happiness of others, there will be no need to use food, alcohol and so on to comfort yourself.

Know Where your Strengths Lie and Take Control

Have you ever locked yourself out of your car or your house? Are you still beating yourself up over it or have you pretty much moved on? You've probably pretty much moved on. Why? Because you've learned to keep your – your *what?* – with you. Hint: it begins with a 'K'! You've learned to keep your *Keys* with you![54] So, you've learned something which can serve you in the future and prevent you from making the same mistake again.

Whenever you overcome difficult circumstances, you are better equipped for the future. Every experience brings you powerful knowledge – tools to help you to progress in life. Add these tools to your natural strengths and abilities, and the result is a very powerful mix which can drive you forward to great things. Ability, learning, experience and the desire to better yourself – wow! It's a mix that can power you forward through thick and thin.

'But,' I hear you say, 'what *are* my natural strengths and abilities? How do I find them?'

Well, you already *know* what they are, don't you? Our unconscious mind knows the truth about our abilities. The White House intern who lost her way and is now a drug addict (and that's a true story) *knows* how smart she really is and how much potential she really has – *she's just chosen to ignore it.*

So, here's an exercise you can do to *reconnect* with what's great about yourself. Whether or not you've already done it in the course of this book, it's a powerful exercise, so do it again!

Set yourself a time limit of 15 minutes.

Now write a list of 15 non-achievement-related great things about yourself. Note the 'non-achievement-related' bit: these aren't about what you've *done*, but about what you *are*!

If you feel blocked, push through and find something to write – anything! For example, the colour of your eyes, or the fact that you love to dance, or the fact that you love your children...

Once you've written 15 great things about yourself, add 5 more so the total comes to 20.

Did you notice that you just took control of your own self-esteem there? So how about taking control of your destiny and finding a way to move forward? When are you going to start? Steve Linder says, 'Step forward or leave those who need you waiting!' That includes yourself, by the way! Don't ever leave yourself waiting to achieve your potential.

Lastly, never compare yourself with others. What works for others may not work for you. As my English grandmother used to say, 'Other people are a different kettle of fish!' So tailor your methods to your own pace and your own abilities and celebrate your individual and unique successes along the way!

Broaden and Build

Positive emotions like happiness, interest and excitement broaden the mind by encouraging exploration and variety in thought and action. In contrast, negative emotions prompt narrow and restrictive behaviour.

Can you remember a time when you were reluctant to try something new but did it nevertheless and were so grateful that you did because you learned something new, met someone new or had a great new experience that really added value to your life?

Can you remember a *specific* time? As you go back to that time, go right back to that time now ... float down into your body ... and see what you saw, hear what you heard, and feel all the feelings ... isn't it great to experience and explore, to expand your world?

Donald Trump urges people to 'Think Big!' You can 'Think Big!' too! Set your sights and your aims high and your unconscious mind will help you to achieve your vision. So, if you want to lose 5lb, aim for 8lb or 10lb. If you want to make a million pounds, why not make that a few million? If you want to serve the people around you, how about doing something to serve the community, society or even the world? If I want to sell 25,000 books, for example, how about making that a million? (Will you help me, readers? Recommend this book to your friends and neighbours, your work colleagues and even your enemies – who'll be grateful for it and treat you more nicely as a result! You'll be part of what my friend Dr. Isaac Jones calls 'The New Health Model' movement: and personally you'll be helping to improve the world: wow! If you are interested in joining us, you can find out more by e-mailing support@designerhealthcenters.com and referencing this book.

The more you stretch your visions, the more likely you are to succeed because, remember, your unconscious mind doesn't know the difference between what's real and what's vividly imagined!

Be Grateful

...for small mercies, big mercies and all mercies! Gratitude focuses the mind on what *we have* instead of what we don't have. When we appreciate what we have and enjoy the simple pleasures of life, our mood is brightened and our brain is gradually trained to see the positive.

So, celebrate small successes – remember that on a journey of many miles, every step counts. Success is only the cumulative effect of many small achievements: in weight loss, in the pursuit of fitness, in career progression and in life. So be grateful for those small steps along the road to success!

Key Points to Remember
- Focus on what you can achieve in the here and now.
- Engage your senses to enjoy and savour what you have and what you can do for yourself (instead of what you don't have).
- Know your strengths and weaknesses and take control.
- Use support where you can, to help you along.
- Add value to others – in serving others you'll be serving yourself!
- 'Think Big!' like Donald Trump – stretching your vision of what you can achieve will help you to achieve it.

- Bolster your positivity every day by being grateful for what you have.

Key Number Twenty-Seven

Move, Move, Move your Body!

It stands to reason that moving your body will get you trimmer and fitter, but how about happier? In fact sporty activities aid the release of endorphins, the so-called 'happiness hormones'. These are the chemicals released by the pituitary gland in response to stress or pain, so they minimize the discomfort of exercise and make it more pleasurable. This is why sport can give you a 'lift': endorphins are associated with a feeling of euphoria!

If that's not enough motivation to boogie on down, then how about the old chestnut of using up energy and, as a result, burning fat? Basically the more you move, the more energy you'll consume in the form of calories. (Incidentally, calories are not, as is commonly understood, a unit of food value: 'kilocalories' are a unit of energy, representing the heat expended by your body using up its fuel. The word 'calorie' comes from the Latin words for 'heat', *calor* and *caloris*.)

What's more, exercise increases your muscle mass and tones it, adding muscle density rather than volume (unless you're body-building). Muscle burns more calories than fat does, even at rest, which means the more exercise you do, the more fat you burn – even while you sleep!

During the first 20 minutes or so of vigorous exercise, your body is burning its reserves of blood sugar as well as sugar stored in the liver. It then burns its reserves of glycogen stored in the muscles. After more than 20 minutes, it starts to use its fat reserves (so-called 'adipose tissue') for energy, and after more than half an hour it starts to tap into triglyceride (blood fat) reserves: basically, you turn into a fat-burning machine!

Also, for an hour or so after exercise, your metabolism will still be racing and fat-burning (as long as you don't have sugary snacks straight after exercise, which will switch the body back to burning sugar and carbohydrates for energy).

As part of a weight-loss programme, ideally you should be doing 20 minutes or more of moderately intense aerobic exercise several times a week. This means continuous endurance exercise which works the heart and lungs – exercise like jogging, swimming and biking. On the other hand, 'anaerobic' exercise – short intense bouts like sprinting or weight-lifting – is not effective for fat-burning (though it does strengthen muscles and increase the metabolic rate, the rate at which your body burns its fuel). As a general rule, the more oxygen you are taking in over a sustained period, the more effective fat-burning will be.

The UK National Health Service now advises half an hour of moderate exercise five times a week. This type of exercise would use up approximately 150 calories per session. If you exercise in the cold, you will increase your fat-burning capacity, as the body uses extra energy to keep warm. Note that if exercise feels uncomfortable, you are possibly moving into the zone of anaerobic exercise instead of aerobic exercise – if you jog, for example, you should be able to carry on a conversation or able to sing along on your iPod!

Alas, many people take up exercise programmes or gym subscriptions only to give up on them a few months later. That's not you, of course! That's because if increased movement or exercise is to be part of your lifestyle from now on, it must suit you and fit your character – so, if you can't bear the great outdoors, there's no point jogging in the rain! It must also fit nicely into your schedule, so it's sustainable, and most of all it has to be relatively easy and pleasurable. When I say 'easy', I don't mean that you'll be taking it easy, but that the pain versus the gain tips towards the gain. The benefits – both perceived and real – have to outweigh the 'sacrifice'. Actually, there's no sacrifice at all when you discover the true nature of exercise: it picks you up, firms you up and makes you feel fantastic!

Before you start on an exercise programme, be careful what you imagine. Many people can only picture gruelling gym sessions or jogging through the rain: that's more than enough to get them curled up on the sofa with a hot chocolate to hand and more pounds around the waist or hips! Instead, how about enjoying the feeling of limbering up at the gym? Gliding through the water on a refreshing swim? Enjoying the peace and fresh air of a stroll? Or merrily setting off gently round the block in the spring sunshine for a jog to run off your inertia and those extra calories, listening to the birds as you feel the breeze on your cheek and feel your limbs relax and your energy rise?

But really the rule is: *never try to imagine how exercise might be, just try it!* What many people do is sabotage their good intentions by raising the bar too high, matching their expectations to what they think society expects from someone who is taking up exercise. Actually, you don't *need* to spend money joining fancy gyms or swimming pools and huffing and puffing on exercise bikes. Nor do you need to do aerobic workouts wrapped in shrink-wrap type clothing, or take up the latest Californian exercise craze, or even dress head-to-toe in designer gear! There's no need, either, to force yourself to take up gym membership if you find the whole scene far too claustrophobic and boring.

I cancelled my gym subscription and deciding to jog around the local leafy areas and parks instead (saving enough in the process for a nice little luxury break every year). But you don't even need to jog to start off with – I began with a few good old walks to the shops every week, running up and down the stairs every day, a few stretches in my pyjamas before breakfast and (most importantly) avoiding couch potato behaviour.

Anything that gets you moving is a great start! For homebodies, how about unloading the dishwasher or washing machine at record speed, or bending down low to pick up all those children's toys? These activities are all great muscle toners. And once you start to do everyday activities with an energetic frame of mind and a bustling attitude, you'll immediately feel fitter than the day before – and the fitter you feel, the more you can start to integrate more sustained movement into your lifestyle day by day.

Swimming is the best entry route to an exercise programme. It encompasses all the major muscle groups and puts less strain on the limbs, as they are buoyed by the water. It tones the body and can provide an excellent cardiovascular workout, strengthening the heart muscles and improving the delivery of oxygen to different parts of the body.

And please don't panic about your shape in a swimming costume. If you start to swim regularly, your figure will soon start looking better and better – and after all, the point here is not to pretend there isn't room for improvement, but to get on with the job!

Exercise becomes more addictive the more you do it, so the best way to begin to love it is to start slowly by being more active at home. Then, by going for walks or swimming or gently jogging, you'll be incorporating movement into your life in a non-challenging way. Once you start to love the feeling it gives you, you'll naturally want to do it more, and you'll be ready to take it to the next level. Remember the more you do, the easier it will feel. The more you put in, the more you will get out. It's a simple (and satisfying) equation.

You can also become truly motivated by visualizing what you want to achieve. Remember to make the images big, bright and bold and see them consistently in your mind's eye. Then all you require is action. Again, make it consistent – small steps on a regular basis can achieve miracles!

For more on exercise, see *'The Benefits of PHA Exercise'* in Chapter 5.

Remember, it's never too late to invite the benefits of exercise into your life!

Key Points to Remember
- Movement will definitely help you to lose weight and keep it off.
- The more you move your body, the more you'll feel good and want to keep fit.
- Fall in love with being active by starting slowly and with something you enjoy, however simple the activity, then build up your stamina.
- The more you do, the easier it will feel. The more you put in, the more you will get out.
- Keep your motivation up by visualizing what you want to achieve and take small, consistent steps in that direction.
- It's never too late to invite the benefits of exercise into your life!

Key Number Twenty-Eight

Sit *Down*!

This one's especially for busy parents, hard workers and people on the go like you and me! Fact is, when you eat food on the run, you barely register it. You will also be less satisfied. That's why when we eat while on the phone, or watching TV, or tapping away on the computer, it doesn't fill us up half as well, or give us half as much satisfaction as the same amount of food eaten sitting down at a table, when we're directing our full attention to the meal and really engaging with the experience. So, sit *down*!

Can you think of five times you've eaten something recently on the run, or in a rush, or absent-mindedly instead of sitting calmly? Write these occasions down now. And write down what it was that was distracting you from giving the food your full attention.

Did you come up with five? If you didn't, were you being totally honest with yourself?!

Standing up doesn't relax the body enough to enable you to concentrate on your food. By moving around too much, you'll also risk indigestion. The only way to truly concentrate on the taste and texture of what you're eating – and to eat it slowly enough to communicate to your brain and stomach that you're actually satisfying your hunger – is to eat while relaxed. And that means quietly, with attention, and preferably in a comfortable sitting position.

Remember the old image of the shepherd having his picnic under the tree? If you've never pictured that, well, picture it now… How does it make you feel? Does it make you feel relaxed? Wouldn't you enjoy eating your lunch sitting there under the blossom of the cherry tree, hearing the birds singing all around you and feeling the warm caress of the sun on your skin, the freshness of the air and the cool refreshing breeze barely stirring the leaves?

Or shall we tell the shepherd there's no time for lunch? Shall we force him to run after the sheepdog while grabbing bites out of a Mars bar instead? How about making him round up his animals with a packet of crisps in his hand, absent-mindedly popping them into his mouth between hollers? Don't you just feel the food sticking in your throat at the very thought of it?

Well, if you wouldn't want to give the old shepherd indigestion, why would you do it to yourself?

Like the shepherd, we need to sit down with our little 'picnic' and eat it slowly. So next time you feel like grabbing a snack on the go, find a shady tree, or a park bench, or a kitchen chair, and eat a proper healthy snack as nature intended. A nice sweet apple is even better than a cereal bar! You'll feel better for it – and you might even notice how nice it is, for once, to take a moment to stop to smell the roses…

Key Points to Remember
- When you eat food on the run you barely register it. So, sit down.
- Snacks and 'fast' food eaten in a rush will not satisfy your hunger as much as a healthy snack eaten slowly and with mindfulness.
- Eating while the body is moving (i.e. walking) can also cause discomfort and indigestion.
- Picture the idyll of a shepherd sitting under a tree, carefully unwrapping his picnic from a chequered cloth and, like him, take a moment to eat in peace and quiet.

3
10 Super-Strategies!

Super-Strategy Number One

Know That You Can Have It!

For a lot of people who overeat, there's an unconscious belief that they don't deserve abundance. The subconscious limiting belief is that they must grab what they can when they can. Some of these people may have had several siblings squabbling over the best portions as a child. Others may simply be compensating for their own hungry lack of self-esteem with an over-the-top hunger for food. In all cases, there's an urgency to consume *now* before it's too late, to finish it all up. There's no balance.

If you overeat, it's because you don't love yourself enough to have the confidence that life will provide what you need. When you overeat, you are using food to make you feel good instead of empowering *yourself* to feel good! You are giving away your power. The 'kick' or 'high' you get from a chocolate bar is artificial. The high you get from inner strength and confidence is real. Which do you prefer?

Now take pen and paper and write this down:

> *'I love myself enough to have the confidence that life will provide what I need. Instead of giving food the power to make me feel good, I will from now on empower myself to feel great and to create abundance in my life!'*

There's no need for a feeding frenzy in the developed world, where obesity is on the increase. Rather than approach food with a famine mentality, we need to start to relax around it and enjoy it in a spirit of abundance.

We need a balanced approach, but unfortunately evolution isn't exactly on our side. Our self-preservation instincts have been honed over centuries of food shortages and our childhood is likely to have been full of encouragement to 'Eat up!' We also encourage weight-loss resistance and metabolic slow-down by embarking on fasts, starvation and 'yo-yo' diets, which the body perceives as a threat. Denying ourselves food when we really need it signals to our bodies that *we are in famine conditions* – which only serves to encourage bingeing, compulsive eating and 'giving into temptation' later on to make up for it!

And when we deny ourselves the nourishment our bodies need on a regular basis, what are we doing? We're simply proving this unconscious belief that food is never plentiful! And what message do you think this type of deprivation sends to our self-esteem?

Now take pen and paper and write this down:

> *'I prove to myself that I'm worth it by treating my body with respect and by enjoying healthy food and a balanced lifestyle with pride!'*

So, think about it – do you really *need* to finish off that chocolate bar today? How about enjoying just a square or two? That way you'll be able to enjoy it over several days and prolong the pleasure! And if you only eat a tiny square a day, and learn to love 70 per cent plus cocoa chocolate, which is actually full of healthy flavonoids and polyphenols, you can even allow yourself chocolate *every day!* Wow! You already know that I do!

When you're able to eat only a square of chocolate and happily leave the rest of the bar in the cupboard, you have taken back the power of choice. You are choosing when and how much to eat. And you are proving to yourself that you can treat yourself (with discretion, of course)!

When you take back the power of choice over when and how much to eat, you realize you *don't have to* gobble up food every single time you see it. If I attend a breakfast seminar where there are croissants and I've already had breakfast, well, there's no reason to eat one, is there? I won't be 'missing out', because here in London I can purchase fresh croissants at any time from the bakery down the road (and in fact my family likes them, so I do occasionally buy them). I know that I deserve abundance in my life and trust that it will be there for me when I choose – there's no need for a desperate rush to grab it all now!

People talk of 'temptation': *'Ooh, I was so tempted I just couldn't resist!'* Well, how about saving your temptation for these occasions instead:

- a celebration dinner at a fancy restaurant when you'll be hungry enough to appreciate the huge choice on the menu
- your own dinner party, barbecue or get-together where you can happily enjoy sharing nice food with friends
- a nice little piece of homemade chocolate cake at your child's birthday party

These are the occasions when you'll truly appreciate your treats! What's the point of temptation if you only half enjoy the result and feel guilty afterwards?

Now you have taken back the power of choice over when and how much to eat, you can allow yourself a small piece of cake or treat occasionally, especially if you enjoy sharing it with your family as part of a balanced diet. This is a far healthier way of behaving than cramming it in just because it happens to be in front of you at a random time of day when you may not even be hungry – now *that's* a waste of both the food and your appetite later on!

Don't forget that our modern lifestyles have much to blame for confusing our natural appetites. Don't be duped! Advertising and social convention attempt to convince us we that we 'need' to eat popcorn at the cinema (we don't – we're there for the movie, remember!), or 'must have' those snacks with drinks at the bar (why? why not wait for dinner?), or 'have to have a biscuit' with mid-morning coffee, even though we've had breakfast at home and are going to have lunch soon enough and all we've been doing so far is the sedentary lifestyle thing at a desk!

Advertisers are very clever at harnessing our natural 'It's there – I'd better eat it up!' instincts by linking food with more and more situations which have nothing at all to do with true hunger or old-fashioned mealtimes. They hope that if they put it there in front of us, we'll eat it up. And when *we* eat it up, *they* gobble up the profits! *We* get fat and *they* get rich. Think about that.

Now take pen and paper and write this down:

> *'I increase my self-esteem every time I take back the power of choice and choose when and how much to eat in healthy balance. I choose to treat myself wisely and with discretion.'*

Here's an exercise to change the way you think about the abundance of food. It will enable you to make reasoned choices based on your true hunger signals alone – not on greed, or temptation, or the unconscious fear that you'll miss out.

Close your eyes, if you can, and you can, and just imagine now that you have an entire store of food in front of you. As you go into the store, see the colours, and the shapes, and feel the textures, and make them all bright, vivid and realistic. Feel the feelings, hear the sounds and fully imagine the aromas!

And now make the colours *even* brighter, the contrasts *even* sharper, the textures *even* more ... textured ... and the sounds and aromas *even* stronger and more powerful. Are you there? That's right.

Now allow yourself to imagine you can choose and buy and eat *whatever* you want. Nothing is 'forbidden', nothing is 'fattening', nothing is 'naughty', nothing is 'bad'! All the food is healthy and nurturing. What was forbidden is now allowed. What was fattening can now be eaten and what was naughty has had its power taken from it. Nothing is bad and everything is good because you know how to make good choices at good times from now on. Now you have the power and the freedom. And you can have whatever takes your fancy, whatever serves to nurture you, and you can show you how you love and care for yourself – how you love and care for yourself and your health, respect and balance – from now on.

Can you see yourself walking around the store? Can you see the slim, vigorous, healthy, fit person you will soon be ... and you are now?

Now put your arms out and embrace your power of abundance, choice and respect. Embrace yourself. Hold that power – your power – in your hands. Bring that power into your chest and into your stomach. Bring that power into your body to fill you up. Embrace yourself with power and abundance.

Now come back into the room.

Give your shoulders a little shake. Perhaps take a sip of water or stretch out a bit!

Repeat this visualization several times in quick succession every day.

By giving food labels – 'good', 'bad', 'unhealthy', 'naughty' – we are damaging the relaxed relationship we should have with it. Only by being relaxed about it can we build a healthy relationship with it – a relationship free from guilt, excess and self-recrimination.

By acknowledging that you can have whatever you believe is best for you, you are accepting the power of abundance and self-nurturing into your life. Life is there to provide and you are there to make the choices that will nurture you.

Now take pen and paper and write it down:

'Life provides and I make the choices that nurture me.'

From now on, there will be no more denial; instead there will be healthy choice. You will no longer be engaging your body's natural defences against famine or eating for 'temptation's sake' or 'convenience' or simply 'because it's there'. For a slim person who eats instinctively, there are no 'blow-outs' or 'I've broken my diet' despair, for there *is no* 'diet'! After all, what are the first three letters of the word 'diet'…?

Remember that there are no 'good' and 'bad' foods to use and abuse to treat or deny yourself, just food that nurtures your health. Get rid of any desperation you have around food – be relaxed, chill out!

You can actually have your cake and eat it – slowly and indulgently, as part of a balanced diet! The more you do this, the more any cravings you might have once had will disappear and you will find your choices will be far more balanced and healthy than you would have given yourself credit for in that distant past. Our body and unconscious mind *know* how to choose what they need best – we just need to give them the trust they deserve!

Lastly, did you know that scientists have proved that cutting calorie intake over the long run leads to increased life expectancy?[1] So, if you eat 'a little of what you fancy', instead of a lot, you may be around *longer* to continue eating a little of what you fancy – now, that's what I call abundance!

Key Points to Remember
- For a lot of people who overeat, there's an unconscious belief that they don't deserve abundance and must grab what they can when they can.
- If you overeat, it's because you don't love yourself enough to have the confidence that life will provide what you need.

- When you overeat, you are giving power away to food to make you feel good, instead of empowering yourself to feel good.
- When you take back the power of choice over when and how much to eat, you can actually have your cake and eat it – slowly and indulgently, as part of a balanced diet!

Super-Strategy Number Two

Think Logically!

Thinking logically means being realistic and, above all, accepting the link between cause and effect. It's being able to deal with consequences.

For example, now you've decided to lose weight, it's logical you might feel hungry or a little tired at times. It's perfectly logical that you might feel various degrees of discomfort as your body and mind adjust to a shift in lifestyle.

Thinking efficiently means realizing that none of these changes are 'difficult', just *different*.

Now take your pen and paper and write down:

'Changes in lifestyle aren't difficult – they're just different!'

When something is different, it simply needs getting used to. There's no magic trick. 'Difficult' is just something you haven't mastered … *yet*.

In fact, now you're thinking efficiently, you'll realize that slight discomfort, or craving, or feeling of hunger or desire, is simply a signal that what you're doing is *working*: the process is underway! 'No pain, no gain', as the saying goes. Remember we talked about the pain of breaking a habit? Pain is a signal that shows you're making progress. And when you know you're making progress, any effort is worth it. So, never be discouraged. To be discouraged is to allow a setback to creep into your plan for success!

Thinking efficiently also means being reasonable and making provision for slip-ups – which do happen, after all. To do this you need flexibility. To be inflexible or unreasonable with a plan risks failure: we've all seen what happens when people make 'sweeping' New Year's resolutions (not you, of course!)

An inflexible all-or-nothing approach (typical of 'resolutions') is not only unrealistic but can also lead to pendulum-type swings in the opposite direction to compensate. Yo-yo dieting, for example, is a (natural) swing between the two extremes of deprivation and indulgence.

Flexibility also means not giving up when you encounter slip-ups or moments when your resolve wavers. Remember in the game of Monopoly you get a 'Get out of jail free' card? Well, imagine you've got a 'Slip up a couple of times without beating yourself up' card.[2] When you give yourself this card, you can forgive yourself a little slip-up or two and stop wasting precious energy beating yourself up! Instead, your focus changes to getting right back on that game board and continuing playing, just like in Monopoly! As long as you're moving in the right direction, a couple of diversions won't change the destination.

The famous American motivational speaker Zig Ziglar has said: 'Failure isn't a person, it's an event.' That's a great lesson. Failure is an unmatched opportunity to learn how to do better next time, to learn not to repeat mistakes.

Now take pen and paper and write it down:

'Failure is an opportunity! It signposts how to do better next time.'

This is why we must never become downbeat or demotivated when things don't go according to plan, but just the opposite. In fact, thinking about where we've encountered pitfalls, what triggered them and how we can improve as a result is a key element to success.

When we make mistakes and adjust our course, we're also taking a longer-term view. This is important because when we're building a new way of being, we need not only effort and a large dose of realism but also time! Remember the first Key, on building up good habits over time? It's the cumulative effort that really counts.

And for those who say they don't have any discipline – don't you clean your teeth every day? Well, that's discipline! Thinking efficiently and taking action is only a habit. That's all it is. And it isn't about being tough or giving yourself a hard time – enjoyment is a vital part of the process. For changes to take hold and become part of your lifestyle, you've got to enjoy them and believe in them. So, if your heart's in becoming fitter, gaining a healthier lifestyle and losing your extra weight in the process, you're already, as they say, halfway there!

Key Points to Remember
- Thinking logically means being realistic and accepting the link between cause and effect.
- It is logical to feel various degrees of discomfort as your body and mind adjust to a shift in lifestyle. This signals that what you're doing is working!
- Thinking logically also means making provision for slip-ups. You can use a mental 'Slip up a couple of times without beating yourself up' card to ensure your focus and energy remain on your plan.
- 'Failure isn't a person, it's an event.' Thinking about where you've encountered pitfalls before, what triggered them and how you could do better next time is a key element to success.
- When we make mistakes and adjust our course, we're taking a longer-term view. Repeated actions over time are what build success.
- And for those who say they don't have any discipline – don't you clean your teeth every day?
- Believe in and enjoy the changes you are making and they will take hold and become part of your lifestyle.

Super-Strategy Number Three

Remember That It All Adds Up

If your grandmother was anything like mine, she would have taught you something along the lines of 'Watch the pennies and the pounds will look after themselves, dear!' I'm sure there must be equivalent sayings for most currencies and cultures. Because this is the best advice anyone can ever give you. And it's not just about money, it's about taking action too.

Warren Buffett, one of richest men on the planet, with an estimated wealth, in 2010, of 47 billion dollars, was walking with Katharine Graham, publisher of the *Washington Post*, when she asked him for a 20 cent coin to make a phone call. (This was before mobile phones.) He pulled out a quarter, 25 cents, but wanted change. She was incredulous! But Warren told her, 'Do you know what that five cents is worth at 30 per cent compounding interest over time? That's *huge!*'[3]

Buffett's a man who has spent his entire life concentrating on how to extract full value out of every asset, and apparently he's as frugal as he is rich! But remember that it's not just cents or pennies that add up; the fact that *everything* adds up little by little. This is one of the laws of the universe and one which we can easily harness to our advantage.

You often hear the old adage: 'Cut that spoonful of sugar out of your tea and you'll lose weight.' Many people can't really conceptualize how one spoonful of sugar can make you lose weight, although they *do* understand that it can make you put on weight, which is ironic! It all depends, of course, on the value you give to small actions. To truly understand that a small effort repeated day after day (after day) can reap huge results, we first have to try it and prove it to ourselves. But instead many people trivialize it ('Oh, what difference is one spoon of sugar going to make?!') and so trivialize the whole process of compounding. Well, Warren Buffet, one of the richest men on the planet, doesn't trivialize very small change, so don't short-change yourself either! Every spoonful of sugar counts. Every action, every thought counts too.

Now I'm not saying you have to give up sugar in your tea or coffee if that's your thing, I'm just trying to make you aware of the *compounding* effect of your actions day after day. If you are forever picking crumbs off your children's plates or snacking from the fridge every time you pass it, you will put on weight: all those crumbs add up! Do you know that if you cut out one biscuit a day with your coffee it will save you approximately a mind-blowing 29,200 calories a year? That means 9.7 kilograms in weight, or 21.4 pounds – a stone and a half! That's the power of compounding.

On the other hand, small actions repeated over time, day after day (after day) can (and do) compound into amazing results. For example, this book wouldn't have been written if I hadn't set myself a small, achievable and non-stressful) goal of writing 500 words a day – that's about three pages! Hey presto, the weeks and months passed and one day I was looking, quite amazed, at a finished manuscript of close to 110,000 words (which was slimmed down a tad later on). As my PhD surgeon friend mentioned, the original length was more than 10 times the length of her thesis, yet it still felt effortless and rather magical.

So, do recognize both sides of the compounding coin. And compounding doesn't just apply to weight, but to exercise and to, yes, as we've been mentioning, your thoughts as well! If you take the lift every day instead of the stairs, you will stay unfit. If you tell yourself you can't achieve what you want every day, or that you're not happy with your appearance, you will believe it – and you will also start to believe that's all you deserve.

But, instead, if you do vow to yourself to take one small step a day, consistently and non-negotiably, to increase the exercise you take, whether it be walking up the stairs instead of using the lift, taking a stroll during your lunch break instead of surfing the internet, or deciding to sign up for swimming at your local pool a few times a week, you *will* find yourself fitter and slimmer in no time! And if you tell yourself every day that you *can* (and *will!*) have the body and stamina of your dreams and the appearance you desire – and you visualize what you're aiming for – the compounding effect of your thoughts will give your more self-confidence and impetus to move forward. Then one day, as if by magic, you'll find your vision is becoming reality!

Key Points to Remember
- Small quantities add up. This is the power of compounding: something used by powerful individuals to create real financial wealth but also a powerful concept you can use to lose weight and to achieve many other goals besides.
- Pay attention to the small quantities of food you might ingest out of thoughtlessness or boredom – they all add up.
- Equally, small and simple positive actions add up. One small step a day can make your vision a reality!

Super-Strategy Number Four

Waste Not, Want Not!

Is your eye bigger than your tummy? Do you over-serve yourself? Do you eat up everything on your plate, even when you're already full?

We live in a world where waste and over-consumption are increasingly a problem. They contributed towards the recent 'credit crunch'. Greed is no longer good – and never was, it's a monster that feeds itself and is never satisfied. And, as we've all learned, it ends in tears!

My English grandmother was the most refined lady I've ever met. She had aristocratic blood, but there had been hard times for her family. She always said that to waste food was a crime. She loved quality – timeless clothes, beautiful possessions and good food – but she never wasted anything. In our house, we stick by her example: we make stock from our roast chicken bones, extra milk goes into cakes and puddings before it sours, we use extra vegetables to make vegetable curries which get put in the freezer for those times we don't feel like cooking. When we go on holiday, we freeze what's left of our fruit juices and stew what fruit's left in the fruit bowl then freeze it, so nothing ever gets thrown away!

Avoiding waste encourages a healthy respect for how valuable food is to us. And the more we appreciate the sacredness of food, the more we develop a balanced attitude towards it, appreciate its nurturing aspects and stay slim! When you over-serve yourself and leave food on the plate to be thrown away, you're wasting it. When you eat it 'just so it's not wasted', you're also wasting it – it's either going into the rubbish bin, or you're treating yourself like a rubbish bin!

The best food habit you can ever cultivate is to serve yourself smaller portions to start off with. As my grandmother used to say: 'You can always come back for more!'

If you constantly overload your plate, ask yourself why. Do you have feelings of want and anxiety? People may call it 'greed', but I call it 'need'. So first ask yourself why you are over-compensating, because any type of excess causes imbalance in your life and doesn't compensate for anything.

If you are used to exaggerating your portion sizes, here's a trick to serve yourself less. The smaller the plate, the smaller the portion, but due to a convenient optical illusion it'll still look sufficient – and you won't notice the difference! At a buffet lunch I will almost always choose one of those medium-size dessert plates for my main course. Of course you mustn't fill it several times over, or it defeats the purpose!

In an experiment, Brian Wansink, PhD, a professor of nutritional science and author of the fantastically informative book *Mindless Eating: Why we eat more than we think*, gave a 90-minute class about 'size cues' – how the visual size of food presentation affects the amount we eat – to a group of students at a top research university, and six weeks later invited them to a party where the concepts in the class were tested out, unbeknown to the students! The result? Those students who served themselves a snack from larger bowls ate 59 per cent more, even after having been made aware of the theory.[4] That's where habit comes in. So, make it a habit to eat off smaller plates, and you will naturally eat smaller portions, and eventually choose smaller plates and portions even without having to think about it.

Think of aeroplane meals. No matter how big the customer, the size of the meal remains the same. And do you think flyers think the portions are ridiculously small? I mean, compared to most restaurant or even home-serving sizes, they are much smaller. But every time I fly I look around and see that most people leave at least some of their food untouched, even when the quality is really good and you get a choice, like in business or first class! If I'm ever tempted to overload my plate, I remember aeroplane portions. If the portion sizes are good enough for first class on the world's best airlines, they are good enough for me at home!

A general rule is to serve yourself a little less of each item than you instinctively want to. Try to give yourself half what you immediately feel you want. You'll be surprised to find after you have finished your plate that more often than not your portion was enough. Remember that you can always go back for more if you are still hungry.

If you really cannot help but over-serve yourself, try loading your plate with high-volume but low-weight foods like salad and vegetables. You'd be surprised the space a few leaves of lettuce take up, giving the impression of a full plate. Do also over-serve yourself by pouring yourself a large glass of water!

Nevertheless, my elegant grandmother always taught me that it is bad manners to overload your plate in public. Whether or not other people really do notice, or care, it's a good rule. *You*, for a start, should care, even if others don't. One thing I can say is that I do believe that if someone's visibly overweight and piles up their plate excessively, other people will notice and think, '*That's* why they are fat.' This thought alone should be enough to shame anyone into changing their ways!

If possible, do not serve yourself when you're over-hungry. Either ask someone else to serve you a reasonable-sized portion or drink a large glass of water (possibly fizzy) before you serve yourself, which will provide you will the feeling of being fuller and prevent you from being greedy.

Lastly, remember that if your eye is bigger than your stomach, your stomach will become much bigger than your eye. And you don't want that, do you?!

Key Points to Remember
- Avoiding waste encourages a healthy respect for how valuable food is to us. The more we appreciate its sacredness, the more we develop a balanced attitude towards it and stay slim.
- When you over-serve yourself and leave food on the plate to be thrown away, you're wasting it. When you eat it 'just so it's not wasted', you're also wasting it – you become the rubbish bin!

- The best food habit you can ever cultivate is to serve yourself smaller portions to start off with. You can always come back for more.
- If you constantly overload your plate, ask yourself why you are over-compensating, because any type of excess causes imbalance in your life and doesn't compensate for anything.
- Here are some practical ruses which can help to prevent you over-serving yourself:
- Use a smaller size plate.
- Remember aeroplane meals: if they are enough for first-class VIPs, they are enough for you.
- Give yourself half what you immediately feel you want.
- Load up your plate with high-volume but low-weight foods like salad and vegetables.
- Think of your pride – it is bad manners to overload one's plate in public…
- Do not serve yourself when you are over-hungry: ask someone else to serve you a reasonable-sized portion.
- Drink a large glass of water first.

Super-Strategy Number Five

Weigh Up the Pros and Cons

Let's have a welcome change of subject now – let's talk about indulgence! There will of course be those occasions in life when you have no intention of being rational or controlled or sensible – especially around the subject of food! However it's always best if before being greedy you weigh up the pros and cons.

Here's an example from my own experience. A few years ago, I was in a very well-known seafood restaurant where the lobster was really famous. You just *had* to choose lobster there! Suspecting I'd never finish a 'large' lobster, I still ordered one. Why? Well, I thought this type of choice didn't come up often, and who wouldn't go overboard on lobster if they had the chance? I decided I'd eat as much as I could and my husband could always finish it off.

As it turned out, I had definitely over-ordered, but so had my husband! He couldn't finish his meal off either. What did I do? I'm afraid to say I forced myself to eat it all up, even though I'd had enough. I could hear my mother's words ringing in my ears: 'You can't waste a treat!'

I felt pretty full and not too good after that meal. That's most of what I remember now about the occasion. I really *didn't enjoy* those last few mouthfuls of lobster – what a crime! And I spoiled my appetite for lobster in the future, because I can't stop remembering how bloated I felt.

What should I have done instead? I should have weighed up the pros and cons of over-ordering, instead of just being greedy!

Special occasions and meals out can all be enjoyed much more when you eat in moderation. If you want to increase your choice, you can still eat less of a greater variety. Just don't eat too much or fall victim to greed. There's nothing that spoils a nice occasion more than feeling sick and overfull – and that applies to alcohol as well as food!

Nevertheless, if you have overdone it, don't despair and don't feel guilty. Decide instead to take positive action by eating lightly the next day or couple of days, so you balance it all out.

Here's an exercise you can even use to turn overindulgence to your advantage! The aim is to create a learned association between the food you've stuffed yourself with and your feeling of discomfort. This serves to nip any future overindulgence right in the bud. Here we go…

Can you remember a time you felt bloated, puffed out and rather sick from having overeaten? Can you remember a specific time? Go back to that time, go right back to that time now … float down into your body … and see what you saw, hear what you heard and feel all the feelings of being totally bloated. Are you there?

Now can you picture the food you ate? Picture it in your mind. Then picture yourself feeling bloated and sick. Picture it as though you are looking at yourself from the outside. Are you there?

Now shrink down the image of you feeling bloated and sick, shrink it right down small and just leave it to the side for a moment, but keep on feeling those feelings.

Now can you see that picture of the food again? Make it big and bright. Blow it up so it too is bloated.

Now take the little picture of you feeling bloated and sick and place it in the bottom corner of the big picture of the food. Whichever side feels comfortable to you is just right. Then I want you to suddenly blow up the picture of you feeling bloated right onto the picture of the food so that it smothers it and they become one. You can make a big sound like 'Swish!' at the same time as the two pictures meet and whoosh your arms widely out too at the same time.

Now repeat it, increasing in speed each time – Swish! Swish! Swish!

Swish! – until you feeling sick and the food are one and the same.

Do this several times, increasing in speed each time.

Now you'll find that you no longer have any desire at all to overindulge in this food – just the very thought of it makes you feel bloated!

Key Points to Remember
- Special occasions and meals out can all be enjoyed much more when you eat in moderation.
- If you want to increase your choice, you can still eat less of a greater variety.
- If you have overdone it, don't despair and don't feel guilty. Take positive action by eating lightly the next couple of days to balance it all out.

Super-Strategy Number Six

Get Enough Sleep!

Studies at the University of Wisconsin, Stanford University and the University of Chicago have found that people who sleep less have lower leptin levels – leptin being the hormone that suppresses appetite, producing a feeling of fullness – and higher ghrelin levels – that's the hormone that triggers appetite and stops you from feeling full. A lack of sleep is also, not unsurprisingly, linked to cravings for higher-calorie food!

Research in Canada used a six-year duration community-setting study to 'investigate the relationship between sleep duration and subsequent body weight and fat gain'. Body composition measurements and self-reported sleep duration were recorded. Changes in adiposity (fat measurement indices) were compared between groups sleeping for five to six hours (short duration), seven to eight hours (average) and nine to ten hours (long).

The results showed that after adjustment for age, sex and basal body mass index, those who slept for the shortest duration gained almost 2 kilograms (4.4lb) and those who slept for the longest duration gained around 1.5 kilograms (3.3lb) in weight (after adjustment for energy intake and physical activity). The average duration sleepers were an average of almost 2 kilograms, or close to 4lb, slimmer![5]

This study provides evidence that both short and long sleep durations can predict the risk of future weight gain. In short, if you get either too little or too much sleep, you risk ending up overweight!

In fact, the less you sleep, the higher the percentage risk of weight gain: fewer than four hours a night increases the risk of sleep-deprivation related obesity to a massive 73 per cent, according to a study at Columbia University, with those who slept five hours a night notching up a 50 per cent risk and those sleeping six hours a 23 per cent risk (after adjusting for depression, physical activity, consumption of alcohol, education, age, gender and ethnicity).[6]

According to lead researcher James Gangwisch, a post-doctoral fellow in psychiatric epidemiology at Columbia University, this is all to do with evolution:

> 'The metabolic regulatory system may have evolved to motivate humans to store fat during summer months when the nights are shorter and food is plentiful, which was a survival mechanism for the body to prepare for the dark winter months when food would not be as plentiful. As a result, sleeping less could serve as a trigger to the body to increase food intake and store fat.'[7]

Not much we can do about that, then, except get more sleep!

So, are you getting enough shut-eye? To ensure seven to eight hours of properly restful sleep per night, try these strategies:

- Have a sleep routine to prepare for the transition to rest mode. Warm baths, light yoga and soothing music are all great for calming the mind and body.
- Good sleep habits include going to bed and waking up at around the same time every day, even at weekends. Ask most parents and they'll agree that their children do appear to have internal clocks that wake them at the same time each day, including weekends and holidays – something those adults without children to wake them up every day at 6.30 a.m. could learn from!
- Jessica Steinitz, of the United States' National Sleep Foundation, which has the catchy slogan 'Waking Americans to the importance of sleep!', says that the body 'does not "learn" to function on less sleep'.[8] We have to realize that sleeping less is *not* a badge of honour or an achievement, and won't

automatically turn us into a head of state or a business mogul (by the way, both no doubt use numerous flights to catch up on their sleep!) Even with a heavy schedule, it is imperative to fit in sleep time, even if that has to include 'power' naps during the day. I once read that the perfect formula for a power nap at work is to clutch a heavy metallic object (like a bunch of keys) in your hand. As soon as you are in deep sleep you'll release your grip on it and it'll fall and wake you, but you'll have had a few moments of deep sleep without fear of being found by your boss with your mouth open and your head on the desk!

- If you hit the sack later than usual, don't sleep in more than two hours past your usual wake-up time. It will confuse your body clock and disrupt your schedule.

- At home, use that DVD recorder and record your late-night TV to watch at a reasonable time.

- Use ear-plugs and eye-covers to sleep if you've got distracting noise and light (while travelling, for example). Dimmer lighting, or dimmer switches, in the bedroom and bathroom also help to prepare the body and mind for sleep. Conversely, switch on your bedside lamp as soon as your alarm goes off in the morning to help you to rise.

- Ensure your bedroom is the right temperature. Too hot and too cold will both impact on your quality of sleep. As with clothes, layered bedding is best: covers that you can adjust and kick off if necessary are better than one thick duvet or quilt. Fresh air is good, however, so do try to keep the window open a crack, even in winter, if you can (but not if you'll be worried all night long about security). In any case, cooler is better than warmer.

- Invest in a decent and supportive mattress covered with natural fibres – despite the expense, it's the single most important aspect of your bed – and change it every five to seven years, or earlier if it shows signs of wear. Turn it frequently. 'Memory Foam' mattresses are to be treated with caution: these can potentially 'off-gas' harmful toxins, and the body is most vulnerable to these when it is recharging and regenerating itself during sleep. Old-fashioned mattresses are a better choice.

- According to Master Neurostrategist Steve Linder, we sleep in one and a half hour stretches of deep REM sleep interspersed with returns to lighter consciousness, so time your wake-up to coincide with one of these and you'll be naturally refreshed.

For example, if you go to sleep at 11 p.m., set your alarm for 6.30 a.m. (Do time the intervals from the time you estimate you'll go to sleep, though, and not the time you go to bed.)

- Before bed, avoid stimulants like caffeine, cocoa, hot chocolate, alcohol, tea and even artificial soda drinks which may contain caffeine without you realizing (these aren't great for your health or figure, anyway). Heavy meals which are difficult to digest or too sugary are also not recommended if you don't want your digestion interfering with your sleep. Dr Isaac Jones suggests not eating for at least an hour and a half before bedtime – sound advice!

- Reserve the bedroom for sleeping and, er, other sleep-inducing natural physical activities! That means *no* TV or computers in the bedroom, though relaxing music may help as long as it is timed to go off once you are asleep. Reading in bed is also something to be wary of: scary thrillers or stressful career reports aren't the best relaxants! The same goes for movies or TV programmes you might be watching just before bedtime: avoid anything with strong emotional content.

- If you find you cannot sleep, get up and engage in something restful but repetitive in dim light, like reading non-stimulating subject matter or listening to relaxing music, until you feel sleepy again. Don't stay in bed stressing that you can't sleep – you'll create unhelpful associations between wakefulness and bed!

- Don't exercise too close to bedtime – at least three hours beforehand is a safe bet. Lighter forms of, ahem, bedtime exercise are of course to be favoured!

Key Points to Remember
- Extensive research now links lack of sufficient sleep to weight gain, excess hunger and cravings for higher-calorie food, so get your beauty sleep!
- See above for some great strategies for having a good night's sleep.

Super-Strategy Number Seven

Trust your Body

My two children love sweets, ice-cream, desserts and chocolate! Aged seven and five, they are old enough to know they like these foods, but not old enough to crave them. In my family we don't withhold sweet treats, nor do we eat them in excess, so to the children they are just another type of food. When my children are full, they stop eating, even if there's still food left on the plate – and even if that food is chocolate cake, ice-cream or dessert! *They understand instinctively that being full means you don't eat any more!*

From birth, humans and animals have the ability to know just how much to eat. Early on, of course, they don't have a choice of *what* to eat, having to accept what the mother provides. Between the ages of seven and nine, the human 'critical faculty' is developed and at this point children very often make loud (and critical!) food choices. But never fear, parents, because children have to be offered a new food on average 11–15 times before they'll start to accept it – which is a protective natural instinct rather than always their fault. And, as many parents realize with astonishment, even school-age kids left to follow their own compasses and make their own food choices are likely to make 'mostly sound food choices and, better yet, they won't be saddled with the weight of the food- (and diet-) related anxiety that plagues so many of us'.[9]

In fact, both anecdotal and empirical evidence seems to confirm that if children are brought up eating wholesome natural foods as well as being allowed small numbers of treats on a regular basis, then they seem to be able to regulate their intake of the more sugary and fatty foods *without* craving them or eating them excessively. All children love their birthday cake, but take a look at the paper plates after a children's party and see how many pieces of cake (and icing) there are left. Very few, if any, on the adults' plates, but quite a few on the children's – and I've been to quite a few children's birthday parties in my time, probably over 150 at this stage, which seems a reasonable number for research purposes!

So, what changes between childhood and adulthood? Unfortunately, by the time we are adults, we tend to ignore nature's cues. We don't wake up naturally, but to the beeping, pinging, buzzing and general annoyance of alarm clocks. We dupe our reproductive systems with various pills. We don't take as much physical exercise as nature intended. And we overeat.

Actually, children aren't totally immune either. Childhood obesity is sadly on the increase and children's natural ability to regulate food choices is being duped by fast foods high in sugar, salt and fat, leading to overeating.

Also, many parents unwittingly train their children's instincts for healthy eating out of them. By telling them 'You won't get your dessert if you don't eat up your main course' they are rewarding them for overeating by letting them overeat even more! By fixing portions and forcing children to finish their food or to eat foods they dislike, they are also taking away their ability to self-regulate both how much they eat and what they eat. And by using sugary treats as a prize for good behaviour, they are associating sweets with comfort and reward – and risking programming their children for comfort eating later in life. This well-intentioned parental behaviour – often based on childhood patterns – overrides kids' natural hunger cues and sabotages the innate moderation that most pre-schoolers show at mealtimes.

Other factors affecting children's food intake include parental anxiety about parenting satisfaction and performance, cultural expectations, parent–child power struggles and even parental depression.[10]

Since you are reading a book about losing weight, it's possible that you too encountered many of these pressures as a child and that they are still affecting your behaviour. Whereas the dinner table becomes a 'battleground' when parents exert control over the child's eating 'for their own good', dieting is the opposite side of the coin once we reach adulthood: the battle and control are still there, but now they are about *not* eating instead of eating!

As adults, we've had many years of experience of tricking our bodies into eating more than we require. What starts off as eating for psychological reasons, to please our parents, soon turns into conditioning, habit and, yes, even physical necessity. Because when we overeat regularly, our stomachs become artificially used to holding more, making it a physical necessity to overeat just in order to fill ourselves up! In obese individuals, this can have evolved to excessive proportions, necessitating stomach bands or stapling to decrease the size of the stomach. Next time you feel like cramming that last piece of cake or roast meat into an already full stomach, ask yourself if you really want to stretch your poor stomach out of proportion, like a balloon.

But all is not lost! Stomachs (and habits!) are flexible – whatever we've learned in the past, we can 'unlearn' it now. Remember that we can 'rewire' the brain! With concentration and awareness and the repetition of a new habit – just as we discussed in the very first Key in this book – we can get back to basics and follow our true hunger signals, and make this behaviour sustainable for life. And by learning to trust our body again, we'll learn to trust ourselves more – and grow in self-esteem as we do!

Think of babies learning to walk. It's only by having the freedom to crawl, pull themselves up, fall over again, try to get those little legs underneath and push, grab onto the chair and get a sense of balance – in other words by trial and error – that our little ones learn. The process of relearning to trust our appetite is actually very similar. It's only by listening to our true appetite – hunger, *not* greed, and need, *not* want – that we can understand and control our hunger signals and satiety. By allowing ourselves the freedom to *feel* and *understand* the difference between hunger and greed, and the difference between need and want, we can finally learn to recognize greed, cravings and psychological 'hunger' sparked by boredom, frustration, loneliness and so on.

You need to give yourself the freedom to trust yourself. Trust that your own body *does* have the innate knowledge to find its own balance, if only you'd give it the chance. Your instincts are right when they tell you that it's imbalanced to eat that bag of doughnuts or that entire chocolate bar, or to drink too much alcohol, or to snack when you don't need the energy. Trust your body, listen to your instincts.

Write it down now:

> '*I give myself the freedom to trust myself, and to trust that my body knows its own balance. I vow from now on to listen to my instincts.*'

Just imagine if a baby were confined to a certain area with no variety of physical objects or space around it. It would find it much harder to pick up the experience necessary to learn how to walk! And so it is with our appetites. Force them into submission with diets and restrictions, punish them with unpalatable choices, and they become skewed so that hunger cues are no longer clear. This is why conventional restrictive diets and regimes, and all that nutritional mumbo-jumbo dividing nutrition into 'good' and 'bad' foods, is self-defeating.

So, it may seem contradictory (Neurostrategists like myself adore anything contradictory, because it forces you to think differently!), but the *very first step* towards being the healthiest weight for your physique is to give your appetite free rein for a few weeks. You are no longer a child faced with pressure from your parents. You now have a choice of what, when and where to eat. That's right! Give your inner child the chance to make the correct, wise food choices!

Turn to yourself and say:

> *'Finally my body and mind and Self are free to make healthy, empowering food choices! Remember how, as a young child, instinct gave me the perfect healthy body? I still have that instinct. Let's allow it freedom to speak its wisdom, after so long in silence!'*

And now write it down.

During this period of dietary freedom, listen to your body and note carefully how it feels to be both hungry and full. Take note of whether you are enjoying your food or not, what satisfies you and what doesn't. These are all valuable lessons you are learning.

Concentrate on the feeling you get when you are *truly* physically hungry – it manifests itself differently for different people. Note also that true hunger creeps up gradually – not suddenly when you pass a cake shop!

It is by learning to eat *only when you are truly hungry,* by allowing your body to time this to regular meal times and by putting a balanced framework of eating nutritious foods in place that you will lose weight and keep it off permanently with very little true effort. Nothing else works.

The key points for your new instinctive eating are:

- *Freedom:* allow yourself the freedom to eat what your body suggests when it suggests it. (Note we are talking specifically about your body here, *not* your greed or your whim when passing that ice-cream parlour!)
- *Get in touch with your appetite:* recognize and follow your true hunger signals.
- *Eat slowly:* take time to appreciate the sensory experience represented by your food – and that means not multi-tasking whilst you are eating, and no TV or strolling or standing up or typing on the computer!
- *Quality over quantity:* a few premium crisps, for example, instead of a whole packet of tasteless economy ones.
- *Variety:* is the spice of life, so enjoy it!

And, above all, enjoy discovering the world of eating instinctively and enjoy the food that nurtures you!

Please keep a food diary or journal daily during this time. This is *non-negotiable* if you want to get the most out of this exercise. Write it at the end of the day, not obsessively, and review it once a week. You may be surprised at what it reveals!

Include all of the following:

- 'What did I eat today? What did I enjoy most? How did I feel?'

- 'Did I eat consciously? Did I stop when I was full? Did I take time to savour the flavours, textures and aromas of the food I ate? How long did my meal last? How do I feel about my eating today?'
- 'Did I drink water? How often, how much and when? Did I drink anything else? How did that make me feel?'
- 'Did I take any exercise today or move my body? How did that make me feel?'
- 'What did I learn today?'
- 'What's one great and positive thing about today? What's another? And a third?'
- 'What was one challenge today? What did I learn from it? How will I overcome it next time? How is this challenge in fact a gift?'
- 'What was new for me today?'
- 'What am I grateful for today?'
- 'What am I looking forward to doing or feeling tomorrow? And in the future?'
- 'Who was I today and who am I looking forward to being tomorrow? And in the future?'
- 'Who did I serve positively today and who will I serve positively tomorrow?'
- 'Who did I show love to today?'
- 'Who must I respect most to optimize my health and my life? Who must I love?'

After a few weeks of this, you will be surprised to find yourself eating far more healthily than you may have expected. Given free rein, your body actually *won't* feel like eating chocolate for breakfast, lunch and dinner. You can now give yourself the credit for making great choices!

A Note of Caution

I don't condone the expression 'ideal weight'. Your ideal weight is simply your healthiest weight – the healthiest, most natural default weight for the average person who doesn't overeat, does a standard amount of physical movement and has no medical conditions which could affect body weight.

The danger in using the label 'ideal' weight is that it may encourage aspiring to a super-thin celebrity physique, which is often obtained artificially through gruelling exercise and restricted nutrition regimes.

The body mass index (BMI) is a ratio of weight to height that is generally used as an indicator of health. It is calculated by dividing your weight (in kilograms) by your height in meters squared. A BMI between 18.5 and 24.9 is considered normal for adults. Higher or lower BMIs may indicate that an individual is over- or underweight. The BMI may be interpreted differently in the case of athletes with high muscle mass. Many celebrities' BMIs indicate they are clinically underweight to an unhealthy degree.

Note that your 'ideal' weight must be *realistic* and *attainable*, which is the trim and healthy (but not skinny) shape we can all achieve!

Key Points to Remember
- Trust your body, listen to your instincts.
- Allow yourself the freedom to eat what your body suggests when it suggests it.
- Get in touch with your appetite: recognize and follow your true hunger signals.
- Take time to appreciate the sensory experience represented by your food.
- Think quality over quantity.
- Eat a variety of foods.
- Write your food diary every day.
- Enjoy discovering the world of eating instinctively.

Super-Strategy Number Eight

Take It Slow!

Our sensation of appetite is largely based on brain chemistry. Researchers are continually trying to turn off the appetite signal by administering hormones, but are confounded by the body constantly finding new pathways to stimulate hunger! To feel satiated, the body will gauge the physical fullness of the stomach and the levels of blood sugar and send this information to the hypothalamus gland in the brain. Then hormones are released accordingly – ghrelin activates hunger, while leptin suppresses it. This process all takes time. In fact it takes 15–20 minutes for the brain to change its signal from one of hunger to one of satiation. This is why we can end up eating too much before feeling full and can feel uncomfortably stuffed after eating a large meal. And, as we know, many of us also consistently override these important 'satiety signals' because of greed!

People are often far too busy shovelling food in to notice body and brain trying to relay the signal to stop eating. By the time the conscious mind, busily distracted with fork or spoon-to-mouth activity, or by what's going on around it, has finally grasped the message, it's too late. It's common to overeat to the tune of 5–20 minutes. That's an awful lot of extra calories! This is why it's so crucially important to eat slowly and concentrate on every mouthful. If you fail to listen to your satiety signals and consume more than you need on a regular basis, you *will* put on weight.

So, 'take it slow' and listen to your body telling you that you've eaten enough. It doesn't matter what's left on your plate at this point. My kids leave chocolate cake! Whatever it is, it's better to put it in the bin, or use it as leftovers, than to put it straight onto your hips or stomach or butt – which is what you'll be doing if you're eating more food than you need.

Remember the 80:20 rule? Eat until you are 80 per cent full, then wait 20 minutes for your brain to register that you are satiated.

One important thing to be aware of – and beware of! – is how different food choices affect our satiety signals. Highly processed carbohydrates and manufactured food items made with refined flour and sugar do not add enough bulk to our stomachs (in the form of soluble fibre or protein) to make us feel full in relation to the huge amount of calories they contain. Our bodies were not designed to be efficient in burning off such hugely calorie-rich substances which are so far removed from those found in nature. In particular, foods containing high glycaemic index (full of sugar!) high-fructose corn syrup and other such high-sugar and high-energy sources, cause us to easily consume massive amounts of calories in a very short time without feeling particularly full. Furthermore, the combination of refined carbohydrates (in particular in the form of high-fructose corn syrup) and low intake of dietary fibre has been a significant factor in the steady increase of Type 2 diabetes in the United States.[11] In effect, these substances are duping our hunger signal system, which is why increasingly they are being linked to the modern obesity epidemic.[12]

Avoid these foods if you want to lose weight and keep it off. Replace them with protein and low-GI (glycaemic index) wholemeal and wholegrain products, enriched where possible with oats, nuts and seeds. (Read more about the dangers of refined carbohydrates in *'The Sugar Trap'*, in Chapter 5.)

Eat slowly. Choose foods which encourage – or even force – you to eat slowly. Ask yourself if what you're consuming is fulfilling you mentally and physically. Remember that foods that do not require chewing are often also highly calorific (soft burger rolls, mousses, melting sauces…).

As my mother used to say, it's very easy to gulp down two glasses of sweetened apple juice but much more difficult to eat the four or six apples that they consist of! And by the time you've eaten the six apples, your satiety signals will have had the time to kick in, whereas it's so easy to drink a couple of glasses of juice on top of a big meal. That's just one example. I'm sure you can think of many others. Write them down if it helps.

Key Points to Remember
- The brain takes up to 20 minutes to register that it is full. Try the 80:20 rule: eat until you are 80 per cent full then wait for 20 minutes.
- Eat *slowly*.
- Understand what you feel when you're full – and then stop eating!
- Remember that low-bulk and high-calorie refined foods dupe our hunger signal system. Replace them with protein and low-GI wholemeal and wholegrain products, enriched where possible with oats, nuts and seeds.

Super-Strategy Number Nine

Ride that Wave!

We all know that if you're successful it's going to make you more motivated, and the more motivation you have, the more likely you are to succeed: it's a chicken-and egg situation! But the opposite's also true: it's easy to give up on something when we seem to be failing at it. How often have we heard people say 'I'm so depressed because things aren't great in my job at the moment'? Or 'I'm so depressed because I just don't seem to be able to lose weight'? Failure in one aspect of life can easily seep across and affect general attitude and state of mind. But what many of us don't remember is the flip side: *energy and self-confidence from one thing can create more success in everything!* The fancy word for this is 'cross-contextualization'.

Let's look at two opposite scenarios. Jane is finding it difficult to lose weight. She started by hating herself for having to lose weight in the first place. Now the whole idea depresses her. All she can see are deprivations and restrictions ahead – and that's on top of already being miserable with her appearance! All the negative energy she's producing by being frustrated and unhappy keeps her stuck in a low-energy and low-creative state of mind. In this state, she's got very little positive energy to propel her forward and make progress. I call it being stagnant.

But what if Jane's just been promoted to a great new role and is feeling a surge in confidence and satisfaction? She can now take the self-belief she has gained from her promotion and use it to motivate herself in other areas of her life. Sounds a simple strategy? That's because it *is* simple. And very effective.

If something has worked in one area, if you transpose it across to another area it can work there too. And once you realize what skills you're using to do something successfully, you can apply those skills to something else!

If you feel there's nothing in your life that's giving you that confidence at the moment, look to moments in the past. We've all had occasions when we've achieved a goal or been successful at something one way or another. Even a past learning experience represents success! The more you think about it, the more examples you'll come up with. Trust your unconscious mind to have the answers.

Now take pen and paper and do this exercise:
Write down 15 non-achievement related great things about yourself. Yes, you've done this before. You can do it again. Do it now.

If you think 15 is a lot, you're lucky. Some of my clients get to come up with 50. Fifteen is the bare minimum, so get writing … *now*!

And now you've got 15 great things about yourself on paper, how does that make you feel? There'll definitely be pride in the mix somewhere. Dwell on that sense of pride.

Now, sit back comfortably. Can you remember a time when you felt really proud? Can you think of a specific time? Go back to that time … go right back to that time *now*… Float down into your body … see what you saw, hear what you heard, and feel all the feelings of being totally proud – there! That's right!

Now take this sense of pride in both your hands, and concentrate on how it makes you feel. Pull it in towards your chest, inside you. Now focus on that pride wherever it is inside your body – wherever it is for you, that's fine, that's right – and really focus on how it makes you feel inside. Do you feel good? Do you now feel a sense of freedom, or possibility, or self-confidence? Whatever you're feeling right now is just right for you.

Now picture yourself in your mind achieving your goals, living your dreams… How do you feel? What are the feelings, the sights, the sounds? Think of yourself achieving your goals and see what you see, hear what you hear and feel all the feelings of really achieving your goals.

Now take that feeling. Hold that feeling. Has that feeling got a colour? Say it right out loud *now*. Has your feeling got a sound? Shout it right out loud *now*. Can you say out loud the name of your feeling right *now*?

Now answer this question, out loud:

> *'How long am I going to keep this confident self waiting for me to take action?'*

Now relax and come back into the room.

Now I'm going to share with you another technique, which will allow you to access a powerful feeling of accomplishment anytime you want to. It's an NLP technique called 'anchoring'. You might have heard of Anthony Robbins, the world's highest-paid personal development coach, using it, or, in the UK, Paul McKenna. It's a technique increasingly used by top athletes, performers, celebrities and powerful people in all walks of life to access energy to enhance their performance. It has been used by the tennis player André Agassi and various Olympic teams with outstanding results, and is covered in Tony Robbins' book *Unlimited Power*. And I bet you didn't know that advertisers use it all the time, for example linking emotions from hearing a song to their product, so we associate, for example, ice-cream with freedom or elegance, or even love or sex, instead of fat and sugar!

The formal definition of anchoring is 'creating an association between a specific emotional state and a simple trigger'. The trigger is a unique movement or motion of our body. It causes us to automatically surge into a desired emotional state within seconds. It's like an athlete who punches the air to celebrate victory. If they do this repeatedly over time, the punch will be associated with the feeling of victory in their mind. So if they punch the air at home they'll feel a quick rush too, even though they're off the sports field!

You can anchor that feeling of pride you felt in the exercise you did above. In fact you can anchor whatever emotion represents success to you. It could be pride, or success, perhaps freedom or confidence. Let's, for the sake of a demonstration, choose confidence. You're going to learn how to create a confidence anchor. Follow these instructions carefully:

Can you remember a time when you felt totally confident? Can you think of a specific time? Go back to that time now ... go right back to that time... Float down into your body... See what you saw, hear what you heard and feel all the feelings of being totally confident. There! That's right! Now amplify those feelings – turn up the volume.

And now turn those feelings up even higher. Make it as 'real' as possible for you: make your sounds loud, your colours bright and realistic, feel the feelings as powerful as you can!

And then turn it up even more! Turn it up as far and as high as the volume and brightness and colour will go. Make it all as strong and intense and powerful as you can. And then some!

And now hold all those feelings of total confidence and grip them tightly between the thumb and forefinger of your right hand. Grip them as tight as they will go. Hold the grip as the feelings surge. And as they just start to subside, release the grip.

Now relax, shake your shoulders and have a sip of water if you want – it's important to stay hydrated!

What you have just done is create an anchor by thinking intensely about a time when you experienced confidence. And at the same time you created a trigger – squeezing the thumb and forefinger of your right hand together – which you can now return to whenever you need to recreate that feeling of confidence!

Now let's test it. Squeeze together the thumb and forefinger of your right hand – that's right, feel the feeling of confidence blossom and surge!

What you've created is a neurological link – a link between cause and effect in your own brain, a link that provides you with new resources for confidence and success.

So, do you realize you can now apply your confidence to whichever area of your life you choose? Because now you know how to access feeling confident!

Now turn to yourself and say:

> *'I'm totally confident I'll lose weight and reach my most positive body lightness!'*

Key Points to Remember

- Energy is self-creating. The more negative energy (frustration, depression, disappointment) you produce, the more you will spiral downwards. And the more enthusiasm and motivation you have, the more motivation and enthusiasm you will create!
- Find something in your life (past or present) which gives you a sense of accomplishment and use this feeling to motivate you in other areas of your life.
- Anchor your feeling of confidence so you'll be able to access it easily when you need it.

Super-Strategy Number Ten

Be Comfortable!

We all know ourselves best, and we all function in different ways. This is one reason why standard one-size-fits-all diets are not the solution! Of all the people I've met (and advised) over the years, there are those who've only managed to lose weight on a low-sugar diet, others on a high-protein diet, others on a low-fat diet, others on a high-fibre low-GI diet, others by using a combination of factors, and others simply by increasing the amount of exercise they take or by portion control. Generally people assume that what works must be the food or food types being *eliminated*, but, listen up, what if it's actually the *reverse*? Could it be that what's *not* being eliminated is actually the most powerful factor?

There is only one truly effective way to lose weight: a nutrition plan based on the important precept that no one food group is eliminated for more than a very short period of time. The reason for this is because deprivation creates cravings. Let me say that again: *deprivation creates cravings!* If we're allowed the freedom to continue eating some of our favourite foods, this will allow us to fulfil our tastes without having to go through denial. That way we're less at risk of becoming frustrated, having cravings and then making it all worthless by gaining back the weight lost once the 'regime' has ended. Because, guess what? There should be no 'regime' to end! If you learn healthier ways of satisfying your needs and eat according to your own comfort zone and preferences, you can make it a way of life without ever feeling that you're on a regime or a diet!

When you implement your own choices in this way, knowing that you are serving yourself in your own best interests, you are accessing the most powerful tools for change on the planet: what I call 'self-optimization'. And when you're self-optimizing, you're leaving regimes far behind! You'll be what I call an 'self-optimizer' and what my friend Dr Isaac Jones calls a 'lifestyler'!

When you're a self-optimizer, you'll follow the optimum life, nutrition and exercise plan for your own individual needs – and it'll feel effortless! It worked for me, for Dr Isaac's tens of thousands of clients around the world, and it can – and *will* – work for you too. Consider the alternative: deprivation isn't about maximizing your life at all, and *this is why* conventional dieting doesn't work. We just don't like being 'banned' from what we love or enjoy. The resulting feeling of misery dooms most diets to failure. Success, on the other hand, is all about enjoying the process of making progress!

Repeat after me:

> *'Success is all about enjoying the process of making progress!'*

Now take a piece of paper and write it down.

So, think carefully about which foods and drinks you enjoy most, and also think carefully about what makes you happy. Your aim is to come up with strategies so that you neither deprive yourself of what you enjoy *nor* sabotage your new healthy lifestyle. You're going to eat things you love in moderation, weighing up where they fit in (or not!) with your new self-optimizing lifestyle, and making choices as a result.

Here are seven tricks to combine being a self-optimizer with enjoying your favourite foods:

- *Quantity:* Continue to eat what you enjoy, but in much smaller quantities. And you won't notice you have reduced the portion size by 20 per cent or even 30 per cent, believe me, if you eat the remaining 70–80 per cent twice as slowly… Dr Brian Wansink, in his informative book *Mindless Eating* states: 'As all of our studies suggest, we can eat about 20 percent more or 20 percent less without really being aware of it.'[13] Wow! Without really being aware of it! Were *you* aware of that?!

- *Speed:* When I think of eating speed, I think of public speaking. I was in an award-winning choir from eight to twelve years old, and we often had to sing and read at Christmas carol services in cathedrals with large audiences. It's quite a thing for an eight-year old to climb up to the pulpit in front of a church full of adults and read to them. Sometimes you even had to stand on a chair! I'll never forget being told: 'If you think you're speaking slowly enough, you're *not!* Slow it down *more*, and that'll be the right speed!' Well, it's the same with eating. The more you slow it down, the better, and the more you'll enjoy it too! My elegant English grandmother used to tell me: 'Chew every mouthful 15 times.' She ate whatever she fancied and was slim her whole life long. Chewing every mouthful 15 times has a lot going for it – it will help you to feel satiated earlier, for a start.

- *Atmosphere and accessories:* I've talked already about the importance of eating sitting down with no distractions and of fully concentrating on the taste and texture of your food as well as being grateful for what nurtures you. Remember that simple touches such as flowers on the table and nice glasses and cutlery can sensualize eating, rendering the experience more enjoyable – and remember that using smaller plates and serving dishes can help to control portion sizes!

- *Super substitutions:* Instead of cutting out food you enjoy, you can 'tweak' or even substitute these foods with great-tasting alternatives. In this way, you're maximizing the health and nutrition, but not losing out on the taste. Here are a couple of examples. As well as choosing wholegrain versions of bread and pasta if you really love these carbs, you can further reduce the glycaemic index (sugar load) of a pasta dish by combining slow-burning ingredients such as nuts in a fresh home-made sauce, together with lots of crisp vegetables and lean meat if wished, shunning the industrial pasta sauces that contain so much added sugar. By eating cashew or almond butter on your wholemeal toast, you're doing yourself the same favour – not having to 'cut out the carbs'! And if you love a steaming cup of hot chocolate in the winter, why not try mixing raw organic unsweetened cocoa with a healthy sweetener (none of those little coloured packets; instead, try plant-based Stevia or xylitol) into a mug of organic skimmed milk or soya or almond milk? You'll be avoiding the sugar rush of conventional hot chocolate, and the cocoa flavour of my version packs a better punch too! These are small changes and you won't feel you are giving up pasta, bread or a comforting hot drink. It's also great fun to work out your own healthy substitutions for more complicated dishes! Personally, I love apple and blackberry crumble with custard: a comforting dish from my childhood. My own version uses unsweetened fresh Bramley apples gently simmered with fresh forest fruits and a touch of apple juice, instead of the sugary compote of the traditional version, wholegrain organic oats and chopped nuts with raw cinnamon bound with a touch of coconut milk, instead of the old-fashioned buttery wheat crumble topping, and vanilla soya yogurt instead of custard. Do you know what? It even tastes better than the original and my kids love it too!

- *Balance it up* by reducing other foods which you won't miss so much or aren't that keen on but which might contribute to weight gain. The bread basket in a restaurant is one prime example. Nobody, and I mean *nobody*, really needs mouthfuls of bread when a delicious main meal is about to arrive! Just hold your hunger for a few moments and drink a glass of water instead! By avoiding the bread every time you eat out or at the canteen, you could save countless calories, and remember that around 3,500 calories represent an increase of a pound of weight. For a person eating lunch in a canteen or restaurant every day, simply skipping a standard 140-calorie bread roll (all other factors being equal) would result in the loss of a massive 14lb over a year – yes, that's a whole stone! – and *double that* if they would have eaten it buttered!

- *Question yourself:* With foods that you may love but which are generally not what I call 'optimizing' foods, like chocolate, sweets, chips, etc., ask yourself, 'Do I love myself, my health, my energy, my success and my looks more than this plate of chips? Or do I love this plate of chips more? I can only serve one of the two at a time, so which do I choose?' You may find you effortlessly choose not to eat the chips! But if you simply *must*, there *is* actually a way to compromise! I do it myself at times. It's my special secret. I call it 'the power of three': *just have three bites!* (I use the same 'three-bite' formula for my children when they are trying new foods too.)

- *Happiness all around:* When you eat what you love, with pleasure and concentration and at a nice relaxed pace, in surroundings which allow you to enjoy your food, you will be doing yourself a favour and allowing yourself a balanced relationship with the food that nurtures you. On a regular basis this will discourage cravings, emotional or binge eating, famine behaviour and yo-yo weight gain, and encourage your metabolism to work efficiently. It is also easier for a happy person in a good mood to feel self-confident, and self-confidence in turn can help you to achieve almost anything!

You see that being in touch with your own comfort zone is very empowering! So, aim to fully understand your preferences and your comfort zone and use this understanding to create self-optimizing strategies. This is the twenty-first century alternative to restrictive diets and regimes – aren't you grateful?! Let's do a little exercise:

Take pen and paper and spend 15 or 20 minutes quietly writing down what you enjoy doing, eating and drinking and where you enjoy being. Go into as much detail as possible across all the locations, pursuits and food and drink groups. If you need more time, take as much time as you need.

Finished? Now take a fresh sheet of paper and write a list of the 'Top 10 Optimizing Factors' you want in your life. These are what you aim for with regards to your core values and the quality of life you aspire to. For example, mine include:

To be optimally healthy
To have a body optimally free of toxins and unnatural substances
To have optimum energy for my life and family
To feel and look as young as I possibly can (and be optimally youthful on a cellular level too)
To celebrate the abundance of nature and the universe by respecting it fully
To respect and love myself in such a way as to respect and love

those around me
To optimally serve others and add value to their lives
To leave a legacy
To enjoy life
To fully experience the pleasure and variety that the world offers.
Now these need not be in any particular order (mine are not).
Just write them as they flow.

You can then take time reading both lists and seeing if they are compatible with each other. This is where strategies can start to emerge!

For example, in my case, I love the taste of cacao (chocolate!) so much that I'd feel I were missing out if I gave it up. But in order to fully serve my aim of optimum health and vitality, I choose cacao that's minimally processed and preferably organic and pure with 72 per cent plus cocoa content, my favourite being an organic 100 per cent cocoa bar! But that's not to say that I'd upset my children by refusing a tiny taste of their normal Cadbury's or Lindt milk- or white-chocolate Easter eggs, when they want to share the moment: family is one of my highest core values.

In conclusion, once you've understood the likes and preferences within your comfort zone, you can take time to work out how best to accommodate these into the lifestyle and health you wish for yourself. You will need to cross-reference both to find strategies that fit all your likes and needs. Some of these strategies may require finding substitutions or compromises, but the important thing is that they make you feel fulfilled rather than deprived. So take time to make the choices *you* enjoy, not the ones anyone else tells you that you should be making or enjoying. It's *your* life after all!

Key Points to Remember
- Identify your comfort zone and your preferences. The only successful 'regime' is one which suits your own desires, habits and lifestyle.
- Devise strategies to fit what you enjoy into the lifestyle you aim for. Enjoy eating, with concentration and calm, and you will be encouraging a balanced relationship with food which will nurture your body shape and your self-confidence.
- Being in touch with your own comfort zone and making your own choices is confidence-building and empowering!

4

10 Powerful Food Habits

Powerful Food Habit Number One

Read Food Labels

I am always surprised by how little many people know about nutritional basics. One friend was convinced for years that a piece of Greek feta cheese with a few lettuce leaves on white baguette was a 'lighter' lunch than a thick bean soup with a slice of wholemeal bread. Note: Food 'weight' does *not* equal calories! Here's an average nutritional breakdown of that 'light' lunch:[1]

- *Feta cheese, standard serving size 38g:* fat content: 8.1g fat, of which 5.7g saturated fat. High sodium content.
- *White baguette 50g:* 0g fibre, 30g of refined carbohydrate in a standard 50g portion, total kilocalories with the cheese: 240 kcals
- *Thick bean soup, 1 serving:* total fat 0.5–3.5g on average, 9g of healthy fibre, 20g of complex carbohydrates, 8g of protein, 120 kcals
- *Slice of wholegrain bread:* 1g fat, 3.5g dietary fibre, 3g of healthy vegetable-based protein, 60 kcals

Granted, one might sound more filling than the other, but the fat and high sodium and the calories in the cheese, and the lack of nutrition in the high glycaemic index (converted rapidly to glycogen in the blood,

152

meaning it doesn't fill you up for long) white bread make the thick, filling, warming soup so much more effective for weight loss. Vegetables and lentils combine vitamins, minerals, vegetable protein and fibre as well as an array of wholesome tastes and textures, and they are also low GI, which means they don't provoke surges in blood sugar levels and keep you feeling fuller longer (for more on GI ratings, read on to *'Powerful Food Habit Number Four'*). Cheese can sometimes be a very nutritious choice – when it is unprocessed, preferably organic, and a lower-fat variety – but must be eaten in moderation or it can be very fattening. Feta cheese, despite its fresh image, is exceptionally high in fat. It is best to restrict yourself to about 30g (a thin slice of cheese) per serving, and indeed preferably per day.

So what's the verdict? The cheese and baguette with lettuce is much more fattening and less healthy than the thick bean soup!

It's not uncommon for people to be unaware of such nutritional values. Despite nutritional information being everywhere nowadays, many people are still amazingly under-informed. I overheard someone say recently that an orange juice-only diet would be great for weight loss! Her friend said that she was going to try the celebrity 'cayenne pepper, maple syrup and lemon juice' diet. Not that you can't lose weight on a single-item diet, but you'll only do so for the first couple of days, before frustration, hunger and boredom put it all back on again and you hit the fridge with a vengeance!

It's a shame not to inform yourself in this digital era when we're so spoiled with access to information. It doesn't take a nutritionist to tell you what is healthy or fattening. Absolutely anyone in the Western world can learn to understand basic nutritional values simply by making a habit of reading the food labels which most of our foods flaunt. And it's being made even easier for us as most major supermarket chains are starting to label food as low fat, low glycaemic index, high fibre, organic, nut-free, low salt, gluten free, etc.

The nutritional information on food labelling sets out the calorific, weight and percentage values of the main building blocks of food: protein, carbohydrates, sugars, fats, dietary fibre, and sometimes also salt and vitamin content, in an easy-to-read manner, either per 100 grams of the food in question, or per serving or package. So there's simply no excuse nowadays to plead ignorance. By the way, there's a reason why the best-known fast-food companies (no names!) don't provide nutritional information for their products or in their restaurants. It doesn't take a genius to work out why...

Do remember, however, that nothing is fattening in moderation. A tiny sliver of a favourite food won't actually harm you. A teaspoonful of chocolate mousse isn't a transgression – if you leave it there! Do remember to count it in your daily consumption, however. Remember that every little bit adds up.

However small the portion, do make a habit of checking the label, though, so that you're able to understand the value of what you're putting in your mouth. The more you make it a habit, the more you'll come to know more or less the composition of what you're eating naturally. That's useful, because after all there aren't always labels around to fall back on! From experience, I'm able to estimate pretty much exactly what's in most foods, even in a restaurant, which makes for great food choices.

Being aware of the nutritional content of foods can help you to manage your diet better – I mean by this your everyday diet as well as any weight-loss 'diet' – as that way, you can include all the foods you love by balancing them with foods which complement them: higher fat and sugar foods are best eaten with high-fibre and low-GI foods, for example, as they balance each other out. Use food labels to help you along the way – we can all learn to be food savvy and be our own nutritionists!

Why don't you choose some of your favourite foods today and sit down to read the labels? You might surprise yourself…

And remember that the healthiest foods don't have labels. They're the ones nature provides, unadulterated and unprocessed. That should tell you something.

Key Points to Remember
- There is no excuse nowadays not to be food savvy and know the nutritional content of what we put into our mouths. Most food packages come printed with all the data we could ever require.
- However small the portion, do make a habit of checking the labels.
- When we are nutritionally aware, we can combine 'naughty' or 'fattening' foods occasionally with complementary foods in moderate quantities, and so balance out our energy intake.
- The healthiest foods don't have labels. They're the ones nature provides, unadulterated and unprocessed.

Powerful Food Habit Number Two

Get Fresh!

Do you think that human beings were created to eat what nature provided or to consume food manufactured by machines? Can you imagine where our modern obesity epidemic might stem from? Ponder on this a little and come up with your own answers (and questions).

It stands to reason that the fresher and more natural the food, the more satisfying and fulfilling, both physically and in terms of taste, it will be. Wholegrain and 'whole' foods retain their natural dietary fibre. This is stripped out during the refining of 'processed' foods. High-fibre, non-processed foods are scientifically proven to be more efficient at controlling hunger and weight. Way back in 1982 Audrey Eyton wrote *The 'F' Plan*, one of the first 'diet' books that advocated a higher fibre intake to aid weight loss. Much dietary fibre – contained in wholegrain foods, fresh fruit and vegetables, pulses and nuts – doesn't provide any calories, takes longer to chew and acts like a sponge, swelling in the stomach and being harder to digest, so reducing hunger and even absorbing excess calories (as does the soluble fibre in oat bran), as well as having other benefits for the health of the colon and intestinal tract.

Fresh foods also retain their full quota of vitamins, minerals and micro-nutrients – all the stuff that keeps you healthy, slim, young, fresh, energetic, attractive and, yes, sexy, too! Convinced yet?! But many of us still consume far too many refined carbohydrates and far too much processed food. Why? Laziness? Convenience? Yet what could be more convenient than fresh wholegrain wholemeal bread and a healthy topping, or even fresh fruit?

I cannot really advise that you regularly consume refined carbohydrates or processed foods if you wish to reach and maintain optimum health, fitness and body shape. Even freshly prepared takeaway foods can contain large amounts of oil, monosodium glutamate (MSG, a flavour enhancer not recommended for pregnant women or children), sugar and corn-flour (a high-GI thickener which adds unnecessary calories). The more 'prepared' a food, the less likely it is to help you to be satisfied, healthy or slim.

Of course everything can be tasted occasionally in moderation, but wholegrain foods do offer so many more nutritional benefits.

Luckily, there are plenty of fresh, natural and very palatable foods which are full of healthy and satisfying ingredients and taste so good that they help to fill up our appetite as well as our tummies! Consider for example the following, which now have global popularity: a steaming plate of durum wheat spaghetti with homemade tomato sauce; a lovely plate of grilled seafood and fresh salad; an aromatic curry; a Spanish omelette made from onions, unpeeled potatoes, garlic and fresh eggs; or even a hearty home-made vegetable soup with crusty brown bread and butter. These are all foods made from nature's fresh and unprocessed ingredients which take very little time to prepare and cook; for the most part they're originally peasant foods from recipes handed down through generations. None of these are unhealthy or fattening! Yet many people seem to prefer to scoff microwave-ready meals, oven pizzas, chips, fast-food and oily 'take-out' foods. Well, they can't complain they're overweight then, can they? You make your bed, you have to lie on it, as my mother used to say.

In Italy there's the 'slow-food' movement, which is designed to combat the 'fast-food' trend and promote a leisurely and full enjoyment of fresh natural foods eaten at table with friends and family and a glass of nice wine! Amazing that someone has actually had to form a 'movement' dedicated to promoting what people love most on holiday. But why should we enjoy that kind of thing only on holidays?

It's a sign of the times. In the Western world, we spend too much money on convenience (read: 'processed') foods and too little time on savouring really good fresh food. And our stomachs and waistlines can tell the difference...

You can whip up a fresh salad or a scrambled egg in almost the time you would have spent reading the instructions on the back of a microwave dinner. OK, you get more washing-up when you cook it yourself, but on the flip side, you also help to save the environment from unnecessary packaging waste! And the best supermarkets and delis nowadays do sell freshly prepared healthy salads made from exotic and healthy ingredients, fresh vacuum-packed vegetable soups with no additives, and other organic freshly-prepared meals containing healthy pulses, for example.

There are also plenty of tasty dishes you can make in no time with a pressure cooker or slow cooker (just chop and add to the cooker, season, add stock or water and you simply press the button and wait!), and even a chicken is almost as quick to put into the oven and cook as a ready-made meal. You can buy chickens (and other cuts of meat for roasting) already trussed and prepared in a foil baking tray – that's if you haven't got the time to find a baking tray in the cupboard yourself! Fish can be bought ready-boned and filleted for the grill, or you can just wrap in foil and pop it in the oven for 20 minutes with simply a pinch of fresh herbs and seasonings. If you can possibly afford it, do buy organic meat: it tastes better as well as being healthier! Remember also that fruit and vegetables that are currently in season, as opposed to flown in from abroad (nice to know you're not contributing to global warming!), will have a higher nutritional value and also taste great.

With all these time-saving gestures now included in the price and preparation of many fresh foods, there should be no excuse at all not to buy fresh foods suitable for cooking quickly yourself. Note that free-range and/or organic, as most top chefs admit nowadays, is best for taste as well as helping to promote animal welfare. British celebrity chef and TV personality Jamie Oliver has done a lot to educate the public on the horrors of poultry factory farming as well as pioneering improved school meals. Here's Jamie talking about it on his website:

> 'Food culture in Britain is a topic that has been close to my heart for a long time. There are loads of great things to say about the state of cooking and food in this country, but also quite a few negatives. Brits have one of the highest obesity rates in Europe and are eating more ready meals than ever.
>
> How we prepare our food and the food we eat has changed over the last 50 years. Generations are not having cooking skills passed on to them in the same way they used to, which may be why people are turning to takeaways or ready meals as an easy option for meals. I think it's absolutely crucial to get people excited about cooking good food again, and passing it on to as many of their friends, colleagues & family as they can… With some basic skills under your belt and a handful of recipes, you'll be able to prepare nutritious meals on any budget.'[2]

Notice that Jamie talks about preparing meals 'on any budget' – because good food need not be expensive at all! If you are worried about your budget, do you realize that packaged and processed foods are very expensive in themselves, because you pay for all that unnecessary work and boxing? So, if you want to save money, buy meat, fish and vegetables in their simplest, most natural form. Even ready-chopped vegetables start to leech their all-important vitamins and minerals once cut. Your purse, your taste-buds and your waistline – and very importantly, your health – will thank you for choosing fresh and natural!

Key Points to Remember
- Packaged 'ready' meals on average have higher fat, sugar, salt and additive content than fresh foods – and are more expensive
- Fresh and natural foods are cheaper, healthier, and satisfy the appetite more because real food tastes better.
- Fresh food preserves all its nutritional benefits, especially if you eat what's in season.
- There are plenty of quick and easy recipes out there using fresh and natural ingredients (see *'Sample Recipes for the Whole Family'* at the end of Chapter 6). Check them out and go for fresh and natural.

Powerful Food Habit Number Three

Think Quality!

Do you like premium champagne or cheap table wine? Would you prefer a Prada handbag on your arm or a cheap imitation? Whatever your views on the luxury goods market, as far as food is concerned, eating *is* as much about quality as quantity!

In my student days I lived in Florence, Italy, and we all know that the Italians are famed for their style and beauty. While I was there, new-fangled 'low-fat', 'light' and 'diet' foods promising to deliver that catwalk figure were flying off the shelves. These were pretty much an innovation for food-loving Italians. 'Sugar-free' was another variant.

Did these foods taste great? Actually, they were pretty much miserable and tasteless! Did they deliver on their promise, at least to help lose a few pounds? Not at all! We ended up eating twice the amount because it was so unfulfilling. Artificial sweeteners (which left a taste in the mouth and a craving for real sugar) and various bulking agents were the norm. Many of these undesirable artificial ingredients, like aspartame, years later have been open to controversy.

Did I become catwalk slim? What do you think? Was I hungry? You bet! I may have filled the 'hole' but I stayed *psychologically* hungry. Then, every time we were invited to a big Italian Sunday lunch with heaps of pasta, roast meat with all the trimmings, crusty bread, aromatic wine and scrumptious desserts, I just fell onto it all and made up for all the sacrifice during the week. Some diet!

It is better to choose fresh fruit for a snack, or a handful of nuts (almonds are great), or a small slice of natural cheese. Not only will you know what you're putting into your body, you'll be satisfied for longer. If you give your taste buds what they feel like in a small quantity they will be happier than if you try to dupe them with all sorts of substitute non-foods.

As I've already mentioned, my English grandmother was a big advocate of 'a little bit of what you fancy does you good'. She was a classy lady who only bought the best food and wine from the most expensive shops. She'd say that if you were going to indulge, you might as well go for the best. She never ate huge portions, though. The food was always so good that she was satisfied with less. She never had a huge budget to spend either, but she bought less, ate less, and never wasted food. She always savoured every mouthful slowly, and enjoyed spending time over her meals. She ate mindfully her whole life long, never put on weight and lived healthily until the ripe old age of 89! And you know by now that she loved her after-dinner chocs most of all!

Actually, chocolate is one food where quality really matters. If you taste high-cocoa highest-quality chocolate you'll find, amazingly, that you're satisfied with a very small piece, because the taste is so complex. Cheap chocolate, on the other hand, is so full of additives that it can sometimes be intensely sweet but at the same time almost flavourless: too much added sugar, dried milk powder, dried whey, vegetable fat, emulsifier and flavourings.

It's the same with any food. Try organic cucumbers, wild Alaskan salmon or artisan-baked bread and you'll be surprised at how different they can taste from the ordinary varieties. The consensus nowadays is that organic produce definitely does taste better. And if it tastes better, you'll be satisfied with less – paradoxically enough!

So-called 'diet' foods very often lack the genuine and natural ingredients your body's asking for when you feel like a little treat, which is why these foods barely satisfy either hunger or cravings. Have a look at the ingredients of various 'light' or 'low-calorie' bakery and confectionary ranges in your local supermarket and you might be in for a shock.

Here are some ingredients many manufacturers use in 'fruit'-based biscuits, of the type marketed to be part of a healthy diet and lifestyle:

> 'Fruit paste, glucose-fructose syrup, sugar, dextrose monohydrate, fruit pulp, glycerine, fruit concentrate, gelling agent, flavourings, citric acid, acidity regulators (sodium citrate, calcium citrate), vegetable oil, maltodextrin, dried whey, salt, raising agents (disodium

diphosphate, sodium bicarbonate, ammonium bicarbonate), glazing agent (glucose syrup, dried wholemilk, thickener (modified potato starch), rice flour, flavourings, fruit concentrate (often equivalent to more than 1 per cent in product).'

Does this list bring to mind a healthy diet and lifestyle? As far as I'm concerned, it's visions of scary test tubes, clinical white laboratories and chemical non-foods! But natural and wholesome images such as fit bodies frolicking by the rolling surf or wheatfields blowing in the late summer breeze are what such snacks often have plastered all over the packaging.

So, beware! Always read the ingredients list first, particularly if you have young children who may be very susceptible to artificial additives. Would you give these biscuits to your children to help them grow and play with energy? And if you wouldn't give something to your children, why would you eat it yourself?

So, next time you are shopping, do yourself a favour, and take a moment to check the ingredients before you reach for that 'slimming' or 'low-calorie' food. It may be low calorie, but high in other stuff you may decide you don't want to put into your body.

The solution, luckily, is easy enough: buy and eat high-quality and delicious *real* food and you will find it tasty enough to slowly savour and enjoy – a bit like my grandmother's expensive chocolates!

Times are on our side, with a move back to slow food and organics being backed by many celebrity chefs, including Jamie Oliver and Gordon Ramsey here in the UK, and our own Prince Charles being an organic farming pioneer. Supermarkets are slowly becoming more accountable and have banned many artificial ingredients such as hydrogenated and trans-fats, and many additives. At last consumers ourselves are slowly demanding more quality, better taste and fewer artificial ingredients. And in this post-'credit crunch' age of austerity, many more people are having a go at growing their own produce and finding out just how good home-grown tomatoes and vegetables taste!

I'm not suggesting you bust your budget by buying all organic foods if your household is counting the pennies, just to be aware of quality and what quality means. For example, just by taking a few moments more and purchasing those loose vegetables instead of grabbing a packet of frozen prepared ones, you can often save money because you're not paying for the packaging – and you're eating a better-quality vegetable too, as pre-cut veggies may suffer from vitamin and flavour loss.

Nevertheless, if you can afford to buy free-range eggs and organic meat, then please do, as there is a definite health benefit to avoiding growth hormones, antibiotics and the other residues found in non-organic meat. Also, buy from your local farmer's market, if you have one. If you want to save money, buy a smaller organic cut of meat rather than a larger non-organic one.

Whatever you're buying, choose quality and freshness and you'll get optimum taste, much more satisfaction and often save money too.

Key Points to Remember
- Always aim to choose *quality* over *quantity*.
- Check labels for ingredients and be wary of 'diet' foods: they contain many artificial additives and ingredients which won't make you feel satisfied and which may affect your health in the long term.
- Beware of the advertising messages – always check the labels.
- It is best to choose fresh fruit for a snack, or a handful of nuts, or a small slice of natural cheese.
- If you can afford to buy free-range eggs and organic meats, please do, as there is a definite health benefit and they'll taste better too.
- Choose quality and freshness and you'll get optimum taste, much more satisfaction and often save money too!

Powerful Food Habit Number Four

Do Low GI

GI stands for 'glycaemic index', which is a measurement of how quickly carbohydrates, starches and sugars are converted by the body into glycogen – that's blood sugar. We're all aware that controlling blood sugar levels is really important for diabetics. But did you know that the glycaemic index has recently become recognized as important for weight loss and weight management?

The Atkins diet fad of the late 1990s recognized that low-carbohydrate diets did promote weight loss, but what was not fully taken into consideration was the difference between the various types of carbohydrates.

Nowadays we define foods such as oats and wholegrain cereals as 'complex' carbohydrates. Other complex 'carbs' include beans, pulses, legumes, seeds and nuts and wholegrain pasta. Conversely, simple carbs (white bread, white flour and its products, refined breakfast cereals, white pasta and milled rice; basically, any refined cereal or grain product) have had their fibre stripped out of them by processing and so are very rapidly converted to blood sugar. Plain bagels, white bread, chips and white rice, for example, are all broken down rapidly in the digestive system and converted to glycogen, causing a peak in blood sugar and the subsequent release of the hormone insulin. Now, insulin's job is in regulating blood sugar levels, and a release of insulin into the bloodstream causes the blood sugar level to fall (diabetics must therefore inject insulin to regulate their blood sugar levels). As soon as your blood sugar level falls, you feel renewed hunger as a result of the sudden dip. (As diabetics are also aware, high insulin levels can also cause the body to store more fat.)

The upshot of all this is that the feeling of fullness from eating sugary and easily converted refined carbohydrates doesn't last for very long! Do you remember the urban myth about Chinese takeaway food: that you feel hungry again half an hour later? It wasn't all myth: Chinese restaurant and takeaway food consists mainly of refined white rice and glutinous sauces containing quite a lot of sugar and refined cornflour, which are all high-GI foods causing a blood sugar peak and then a trough, leading to cravings for food even after having eaten a 'heavy' meal. What's more these peaks and troughs aid fat retention. Not good!

This is where low-GI foods come in. Being digested over a long period, they help to keep blood sugar levels stable, to regulate food intake (through the fullness factor) and encourage the body to store less fat. Feeling fuller for longer also helps to nurture a more balanced relationship with food and avoid cravings.

Books rating foods by glycaemic index and low GI-recipe books are all readily available – in the UK, celebrity chef Anthony Worrall Thompson has written several in response to being diagnosed with 'syndrome X' or 'metabolic syndrome', a pre-diabetic state. You might also find reference to 'GL', glycaemic load, which also refers to how differing foods convert into simple glucose, but usefully ratings are based on average portion sizes.

Basically, eating low GI is neither a fad nor a new-fangled diet trick, but simply common sense. If your insulin and blood sugar levels are all over the place, it's logically very difficult to lose weight and keep it off, and a real challenge to build a healthy awareness of your body's true needs and recognize real hunger.

Most importantly, GI 'diets' are not crash diets or one-sided diets and do not exclude food groups which are important sources of nutrients, vitamins and minerals (as the Atkins diet does). The GI diet also doesn't absolutely exclude even 'sugary' foods, instead providing awareness of how to combine the odd (small) sugary snack with lower-GI foods so as to reduce the effect on blood sugar. For example, a high-GI bagel with low-GI peanut butter means the bagel will impact your blood sugar level less than if it were eaten plain; similarly with raisins combined with nuts and cheese. GI ratings, once understood, can help promote a balanced diet where even higher GI foods are allowed in moderation, so cravings and deprivation are no longer a problem The GI system is a common sense system: once you understand the ratings, you choose your own foods. Combined with a reduction in fatty foods and regular exercise, as well as eliminating processed foods in favour of healthy unprocessed and natural foods, it can be a very effective weight-loss and maintenance system for life!

It is not in the remit of this book to go into the details of various the GI ratings, but I recommend that you buy a guide and have a quick read. Remember that GI is *not* a diet plan but a valuable reference point in understanding how various foods may affect our hunger level, blood sugar levels and weight. Like all systems, of course, it is best used in conjunction with common sense.

Key Points to Remember
- The glycaemic index (GI) is a measurement of how quickly certain foods – notably carbohydrates, starches and sugars – are converted by the body into glycogen (blood sugar).
- Eating lower-GI foods can help your body to maintain steady blood sugar levels and thereby encourage stable hunger patterns, discourage binges and cravings and assist in maintaining a healthy weight.
- The GI index is a useful tool to evaluate which foods will affect blood sugar levels most.
- GI is not in itself a diet plan, but a valuable reference point in understanding how various foods may affect our hunger level, blood sugar levels and weight.

Powerful Food Habit Number Five

The Power of Protein

One of the main reasons why people fail on diets is … they're hungry! And the hungrier you feel, the more you're likely to overindulge, comfort eat or seek those sugar fixes which don't provide you with real sustainable energy and which will sabotage your healthy-eating plan!

The trick is to eat food which makes you feel fuller for longer. Several studies[3] have indicated that calorie for calorie, protein fills you up more than fats or carbohydrates do, in effect acting as an appetite suppressant.

The word 'protein' comes from the Greek word *protos*, which means 'first', because protein provides the fundamental building blocks of life, supporting the growth and development of all living things, which is why it's so important to our health and well-being. The amino acid chains formed from protein and peptides repair our bodies and give us essential physical and mental energy.

Protein is digested slowly, delaying absorption into the bloodstream and keeping you, quite literally, fuller longer! This means that eating more protein can help you to lose pounds and control your weight. Protein also builds muscle mass instead of fat, to ensure you stay strong and fit as you decrease your calorie consumption. On the other hand, low-calorie but *low-protein* diets can cause muscle wastage (which is then replaced by fat once weight is regained). Muscle also burns, pound for pound, more calories than does fat, even at basal metabolism – when you are asleep, for example.

The amino acids from proteins are also used to build neurotransmitters (the chemical 'messengers' in our brains), including serotonin, the 'happiness hormone', which improves mood; adrenaline, which needs no introduction; and dopamine, a hormone which is involved with reward and motivation. What better incentive to remember to include enough protein in your diet?!

And the good news doesn't stop there! At a study at the University of Copenhagen, 900 adults and 800 children who had already lost weight were placed on one of five diets designed to help them maintain this weight loss. After six months, *only those on a high-protein and low-GI diet* hadn't regained weight…[4]

Now note the importance of combining low GI foods with protein (we discussed them in the previous Key). According to the *Journal of the American College of Nutrition*, high-protein diets (25 to 35 per cent of daily calorie intake) can aid with hunger management; but it's important to remember that *very* high protein diets (more than 35 per cent of daily intake) are not recommended. Despite the hype surrounding celebrity-endorsed diets such as the Atkins diet, these regimes are not considered healthy or safe long term.

So beware of thinking that eating protein alone can be the holy weight-loss grail: some by-products of protein digestion (ammonia for example) are toxic to the body and in excess can put unnecessary pressure on the kidneys. It has also been suggested that high-protein diets contribute to osteoporosis, because calcium is released from the bones to combat the high blood acidity which results from protein metabolism (metabolic acidosis). In any case, high-protein diets often lack the vital vitamins and nutrients required to neutralize such effects.

Ensure you have enough protein in your diet in the form of one portion of lean meat, low-fat dairy, eggs or fish at every meal (of an amount ideally which can fit in the palm of one hand), but remember to combine it carefully with complex carbohydrates and dietary fibre (technically called 'polysaccharides') in the form of vegetables, bran, fruits, nuts, pulses and wholegrains. Remember that the dietary fibre ('indigestible polysaccharides') in low-GI foods aids satiety, helps to reduce the number of calories absorbed and keeps blood sugar levels steady. A minimum of 25 grams a day of fibre is recommended, which is why a balanced diet is so important, as protein foods contain little or no fibre at all. So in conclusion, protein-rich foods combined with high-fibre and low-GI foods are your best bet for stable blood sugar levels.

Patrick Holford, author of the acclaimed 'Holford Diet', suggests the optimum combination of protein, complex carbohydrates and vegetables in the ratio of 1:1:2 at every meal.[5]

The NPU of a protein, its 'net protein usability', is its particular power balance and usefulness to the body.[6] Much vegetable-based protein, such as quinoa (pronounced 'keen-wa', a grain from the Andes), and brown rice and lentils for example, has excellent NPU, as do tuna, cod, salmon, sardines, chicken, eggs, yogurt and cottage cheese.

The '*28-Day Food Awareness Plan*' in Chapter 6 of this book includes no more than a day or two of lean protein at one stretch, and this only to kick-start the metabolism and induce fat-burning. For maintenance and weight management, however, the whole variety of whole food groups should form the mainstay of your everyday diet.

Key Points to Remember
- Protein acts as an appetite suppressant and prevents you from losing all-important muscle mass, while also burning more calories than fat cells, and building organ tissue, enzymes and the neurotransmitters which relay messages in the brain.
- Eat protein at every meal to prevent hunger pangs and build health and strength.
- Very high protein diets, however, increase the risk of osteoporosis and kidney disease.
- Recent major studies have found that a high-protein diet combined with low-GI diet can aid satiety, keep blood sugar levels steady, and prevent snacking and cravings.
- So the high-protein and low-GI combination is the perfect Lifestyle solution for optimum health, fitness and trimness!

Powerful Food Habit Number Six

Keep a Food Journal

Keeping a journal is back in fashion! Before blogs and TV and before the whole 15-minutes of fame phenomenon, diaries were standard practice: Socrates, the first of the Greek philosophers (469–399 bc), urged: 'Know thyself!' Nowadays, it's Oprah Winfrey who's one of the biggest fans, saying, 'Keeping a journal will absolutely change your life in ways you've never imagined!'

It's pretty logical that writing down what you think, feel and do can help you to understand your thoughts, actions, motives and behaviour. What's surprising is that more people don't take advantage of this valuable tool.

A journal can be so much more than a simple diary – it can be a chart of your progress towards whatever you want to achieve. When you document your ambitions and progression on the page in stark black and white, there's nowhere to hide – you have to take full responsibility and accountability for your actions, successes and failures. It's much harder to twist the truth when you're forced to write it all down in detail. A journal can also serve as moral support if you write down motivating phrases and quotes and add pictures to remind yourself of where you want to be.

How does a journal differ from a blog? The two might be very similar, but with a blog there's always the fact that you're writing with an audience in mind. So you might not be brutally honest with yourself! In a journal, or diary, on the other hand, there's nothing between you and your deepest secrets.

A journal can provide you with a sense of control and can help to understand feelings and obstacles. It can help to clarify plans, put issues into perspective and relieve stress. Writing down your goals and aims also serves to cement them into your unconscious mind. Remember that the unconscious mind doesn't differentiate between what's real and what's vividly imagined, and writing things down helps to produce those all-important mental images. Most importantly, however, a journal gives you a record for future reference so that it's easier to track your progress.

If you aren't into writing a journal, just a few lines on a piece of paper can help. But make sure you keep the paper somewhere where you can see it every day and chart how you're doing. Update it every month or so to reflect developments.

As far as keeping a food journal is concerned, this can help to stamp out bad nutritional habits which you may have been conveniently glossing over or may not be conscious of. You may find you're amazed at the occasions for overeating or overindulging which have escaped your attention, for example:

- Are you consuming too many sugary snacks or too many fast foods or too many fizzy drinks?
- Do you eat a standard amount regularly or do you skimp on one meal only to make up for it at the next?
- Do you skip breakfast? (It's a 'no-no'! Eating breakfast kick-starts the metabolic rate, enabling you to start the day burning energy, so skipping breakfast is a sure-fire way to sabotage an efficient metabolism and steady weight loss, contrary to what many people believe.)
- Do you snack too much between meals? If you have been eating the right amount to satisfy your hunger, one snack mid-morning and one mid-afternoon should suffice (and one piece of fruit or yogurt before bedtime, if you eat a very early dinner).
- Do you constantly 'taste' foods, snap off a little corner, try a spoonful, ask for a bite, check the seasonings, pick out the raisins, pop in a leftover – and think that none of these count? (This is a common pitfall, but all these seemingly innocuous activities build up calorie count very quickly!)

- Do you eat enough vegetables and fruit or overload on the carbohydrates?
- Do you eat a balanced meal three times a day or 'graze' instead?

It's also easier to plan a balanced diet if what you're eating is documented. When you make a list of your daily eating under the headings of food groups, you can immediately tell where the areas for improvement are.

Do also write down your thoughts and feelings, especially the positive ones. By focusing on the positive, you'll find that you're in a better frame of mind to make progress toward your goals. Documenting successes along the way is a great boost to motivation. And because a journal stretches into the future, the longer-term view encourages us to be more patient. Success can take time and effort, but if the process and direction are being mapped out, you've got more motivation to go the stretch!

Your journal will also show you where you might slip up occasionally: valuable information for learning to do better next time! Remember imperfection is a human trait and a setback simply a little stumble, so get up again and move on with a smile on your face!

The most useful part of keeping a journal is the way in which it encourages honesty, so do be honest with yourself and use this awareness to make changes for the better. Do not despair if less than savoury truths are highlighted – this is your own private chance to grab the bulls by the horns! Keep up documenting your progress day by day, instigating changes where necessary and you will soon find you're racing along towards your goal really feeling more controlled and self-confident than ever!

Bob Greene, a renowned exercise physiologist, bestselling author and a certified personal trainer (of Oprah Winfrey, amongst others), advocates keeping a daily journal where each day has a section where goals are recorded (in his case, fitness and exercise goals) and another section where feelings and eating patterns can be recorded. The days are then summarized weekly to provide a snapshot of how clients are progressing and Greene provides quotations to inspire and motivate.

You can use a similar format for your own version:
- a daily section, with space to record thoughts and feelings (you can even split up sections into the different times of day if you want)
- a weekly summary to provide a snapshot of progress
- a comparison of short-term goals (daily) with medium-term (weekly) and longer-term goals (monthly, say)
- a projection of long-term goals for the future (six-monthly, say, or longer)

You can add quotations and pictures to inspire and motivate. Enjoy the process and personalize it!

Key Points to Remember
- The benefits of keeping a food journal (or indeed, any journal) include taking responsibility and increasing accountability.
- With a journal we can chart progress not only via a series of 'snapshots' but also over a period of time, so that we are able to look back over our successes and fuel our motivation.
- A journal also builds patience because of its longer-term timescale.
- An ideal format will include a daily 'goals' section and another section where feelings and thoughts can be recorded. A weekly summary can provide a snapshot of progress.
- Remember to plot your long-term goals for the future (six-monthly, say, or longer).
- You can add quotations to inspire and motivate, pictures and whatever else you feel adds value and helps you to enjoy the process.

Powerful Food Habit Number Seven

Be a Master Chef!

The relationship we have with food will ultimately determine how slim and fit we are. Many people who fight being overweight, whether by a few pounds or kilograms or more, have a love–hate relationship with food. These love–hate relationships are by their nature addictive relationships. I have often heard people say that they feel manipulated by food and have no control over what and how much they eat. These are people who literally dream (or daydream!) of food, and it takes up much of their daily working memory either trying to avoid it or else giving into it. But ask many of the same people if they like to cook, and many say that they don't: they prefer fast food or ready meals!

But the vehicle to a better relationship with food is (as with any relationship!) to spend *quality* time and care with it. And spending quality time and care with food means learning how to cook!

Learning to cook properly – which means not just putting a chicken into the oven or a ready meal into the microwave – teaches us not only about ingredients and tastes and flavours but can enhance our respect for eating slowly and with concentration (which alone can keep us slimmer): there will be less of an urge to scoff down food quickly if you've spent hours preparing and cooking it! And when you're aware of the ingredients, you naturally start to pay more attention to the finer details of taste and texture.

Respecting your health and loving yourself mean giving yourself the gift of nurturing yourself with a great variety of good healthy food presented in an exciting way. You can be proud of cooking it yourself!

Learning to cook properly is also a very useful discipline for those compulsive eaters who cannot see food without tasting it, who cannot pass a bowl of nuts without eating a few and who can barely walk past the fridge without opening it and snacking. (My mother used to joke that it was no point opening the fridge continually, as if something else had materialized in it in the meantime, as she hadn't gone shopping yet!) Although professional cooks naturally do have to taste their wares, cooking teaches compulsive eaters to be around food without – to put it bluntly – having to put it in their mouths all the time (my mother used to call this habit 'picking'). If you tend to 'pick' at food whenever you see it in front of you, cooking can teach you self-control – you can't be forever picking at ingredients destined for a dish, or tasting raw ingredients. Leave the spoon licking to the children!

Put a rule in place when you are cooking that you taste only twice – once for salt or seasoning, and once to see if the food is cooked – which often is not necessary, as texture is a reliable indicator. I have a friend who is an amazing cook. Despite being totally vegetarian himself, he cooks lots of meat- and fish-based dishes for his family without ever having to taste them and they all come out highly professionally. So, cut the excuse that constant tasting is a must – it's not!

Slim people are able to be around food, appreciate its colour, taste and smell, and still not feel an uncontrollable urge to eat it. But many overweight people can't see or smell food without feeling a need to eat it. Cooking can teach a more balanced approach.

When we learn how to cook well, we also dedicate ourselves to learning about ingredients, learning how to shop for them, and learning how to appreciate food for its myriad of wonderful tastes, textures and perfumes. Shopping for ingredients to construct a wonderful meal with time and care is very different from shopping out of greed or hunger. Planning a meal which is a labour of love for you and your family, and sitting down and eating it calmly and slowly and with attention, with the respect due to it – especially after all the effort that has gone into its creation! – can help to overcome the urge for instant gratification which often results in people being overweight.

Cooking in itself brings an element of patience into the equation: you have to learn to be patient around food if you are cooking from scratch. Patience and care and respect around food are all weapons against compulsive eating, snacking and bingeing. The aim is to learn to wait for a meal and then to eat it slowly and with joy.

Remember that cooking need not be a chore or a lot of effort. Simply delicious meals can be prepared at home quickly and easily. For those who are nervous about learning to cook, I thoroughly recommend Jamie Oliver's *Cook with Jamie: My guide to making you a better cook* and *Jamie's Ministry of Food* books, which provide an easy-to-follow approach to basic and nutritious home cooking – of the tasty, good and wholesome kind!

Key Points to Remember
- Learning to cook will enhance our relationship with food, which, ultimately, will determine how slim and fit we are.
- Cooking teaches us to be around food without feeling the need to eat or taste it constantly.
- Shopping for ingredients brings an element of patience into the equation.
- Cooking need not be a chore or a lot of effort. Simply delicious meals can be prepared at home quickly and easily.

Powerful Food Habit Number Eight

Spiritual Wisdom (Eat with Gratitude)

Whatever our faith or religion, we can all learn a valuable lesson from spiritual teachings about food, especially those of the Buddhist school. All schools of Buddhism involve food in rituals, chants are expressed before and after meals, and historically the practice of offering food as alms to monks was considered a very important duty. Hinduism also reveres offering food: again both to deities and to holy men.

My husband's family is from India and I've witnessed first hand just how much food is venerated there. The food given as offerings at the temples in praise of the gods is never wasted. It is referred to as *Prasad* or *Prasadum*, 'holy food', and, after being blessed, is collected and handed out to worshippers. Hindus believe that *Prasad* is full of sacred blessed energy, so it's a special honour to take it home to enjoy. The best morsels are always kept for the kids and this sort of treat actually does really taste kind of special!

We can all learn from these rituals. They show gratitude for the food that fuels us and encourage us to look at food in a wider context. The Christian grace, giving thanks to God for the food we eat, similarly gives thanks to a higher power for giving us food to nurture us.

For good reason, too: food is the raw material to support the growth, repair and maintenance of our bodies! What is amazing is not simply that our bodies are made up of 50 to 75 *trillion* cells,[7] but that many of us really don't seem care very much about how we nourish these cells. (That wouldn't be you now, would it?!)

In the Buddhist Zen tradition the emphasis is not only on a higher power but also on our own human contribution. Reflection is invoked on the human effort which has served us in bringing our food to table. Similarly, a Nichiren Buddhist chant says, 'Even a drop of water or a grain of rice is nothing but the result of meritorious work and hard labour.' It's offering gratitude to the human beings, both past and present, who have helped to bring our food to the table. Food, in its best and most natural form, is the result of organic processes, patience, hard work and husbandry (as opposed to convenience, artificial processing and mechanization). The best food is food where human touch and care have been involved in producing and preparing it.

It is important not to take anything in life for granted, especially the food that nourishes us (think of a starving child to fully acknowledge this truth). We need to remind ourselves to appreciate food for its role in sustaining the health of both body and mind.

When we have reverence for food, we can start to behave differently around it – neither abusing it, wasting it, bingeing on it nor eating 'food' that has long ceased to have any real similarity to what nature originally intended. When you respect food, you give it your full and mindful attention.

Mindfulness is also invoked in Buddhism, and indeed during the Christian 'grace'. As you now know, it means full attention to the moment and is the answer to transcending greed (*check out page 000 and page 000 for more information on how to improve your mindfulness when eating*).

Obese individuals have been observed to reach for more and more food without taking the time to taste what they're actually eating, forking in new food before they've even finished the previous mouthful.[8] There's no mindfulness to this way of eating and food satisfies less (which leads to overeating, which leads to excess weight – it's a vicious cycle).

Theravada, the oldest school of Buddhism, reflects, 'I will allay hunger without overeating, so that I may continue to live blamelessly and at ease.'[9] If we are searching for happiness outside ourselves, we will never be fulfilled. Using food to make us happy – or anything external to make us happy – will never satisfy us and we will continue to suffer craving. Being greedy can only encourage this craving and this unhappiness.

Food can only fill the stomach – it can't fill holes in the heart, mind or soul! It cannot fill cravings for love, peace, security or happiness, whatever or however much we eat.

When I lived in Japan, I noted that no one ever started to eat without saying, '*Itadakimasu*.' This means 'I receive' and is an expression of gratitude and reverence for the food in front of you. The Japanese are extremely reverent about their food, and this reverence, I am certain, contributes to the attention and care taken not only in the presentation of food and combination of ingredients, but the mindfulness with which Japanese appreciate what they're eating. No doubt this contributes to the Japanese cuisine being as healthful as it is and the Japanese being as slim as they are!

Similarly, my mother-in-law, who is Hindu, offers the first mouthful of any food she eats to heaven, to her gods, in reverence.

When we too learn to look at food with a spirit of gratitude, and with a sense of reverence for its nurturing qualities, we learn to eat without greed and in turn become slimmer and happier and more fulfilled, appetite, body and soul!

Give thanks every day for the food you eat, remember the care and toil that were taken in its production and vow to treat it with the respect it deserves. In return, it will respect you, your health and your body.

Key Points to Remember
- Whatever our faith or religion, we can all learn a valuable lesson from spiritual teachings about food.
- When we have reverence for food, we can start to behave differently around it – neither abusing it, wasting it, bingeing on it nor eating 'food' that has long ceased to have any real similarity to what nature originally intended.
- When you respect food, you give it your full and mindful attention.
- Mindfulness is the answer to transcending greed.

- When we learn to look at food with a spirit of gratitude, and with a sense of reverence for its nurturing qualities, we learn to eat without greed and in turn become slimmer and happier and more fulfilled, appetite, body and soul!
- Give thanks every day for the food you eat, remember the care and toil that were taken in its production and vow to treat it with the respect it deserves.

Powerful Food Habit Number Nine

Balance It Up!

Let's face it, when you traditionally think about dieting, do you think about balance? Not only have you got bingeing on one side of the spectrum and fasting on the other, but you've got yo-yo dieting in the middle, wildly swinging from one end to the other. Hunger is counterbalanced by overeating and weight loss is counterbalanced by subsequent weight gain! Not very balanced or harmonious, and not very good for your health, either.

The irony is that balance was precisely nature's original intent: our body and mind have evolved over millennia to prevent us from starvation, balancing out times of famine with the times of plenty, literally in order to keep us alive.

Although most of us are no longer hunter-gatherers who have to overeat when food is plenty as there is no guaranteed long-term supply, many people in remote parts of the world still do eke out a nomadic hunter-gatherer-type existence, finding food where they can. Others rely on the uncertainty of harvest in precarious climate conditions made worse by global warming affecting crop supply. So, since we have been unable to eradicate famine in the world, our body hasn't yet eradicated the natural fast–feast instinct. What's more, it self-regulates food intake through two main processes: what's referred to as 'sensory specific satiety' (when we feel we've had enough) on the one hand, and caloric compensation (when we make up for 'lost' calorie intake, for example after being ill or losing weight too quickly) on the other.[10]

We all know how utterly frustrating it is putting all the weight back on when you've just spent several weeks (or months) starving yourself to lose it, but remember that your body's merely trying to achieve *balance*. It's a survival instinct. But what if you gave your body the gift of balance *every day*? Wouldn't it be happier then?

It's not for nothing that a 'balanced diet' is considered the healthiest long term. So what does that say about diets which reduce or eliminate entire food groups, like the original Atkins diet, for example, where a large proportion of fats and protein were allowed but no carbohydrates at all? Or newer versions of the high-protein regime which exclude even green vegetables or salad? We've already touched on this briefly. These regimes have definitely been proven to cause weight loss in the short to medium term, but anecdotal evidence suggests that people who enjoy their carbohydrates, or even their fruit, are prone to crave these to excess once the regime ends – and risk putting much of the weight they had lost straight back on again once caloric compensation kicks in and the body makes up for lost balance. In fact, for this very reason the original Atkins regime has been modified to include complex carbohydrates in its final phase, and the recently popular Dukan diet's success depends on pretty complicated and stringent readjustment routines, where 'forbidden' foods are gradually reintroduced over a prolonged period of time.

On the other hand, when you eat a balanced and varied diet, without denying yourself essential food groups and nutrients, and eat as much as your body needs whenever it is hungry but stop when you are full, and do so on a long-term basis, you will find that fast–feast 'yo-yo' behaviour becomes a thing of the past! Your body will trust that there is food to be had in the correct quantities and of the types it needs, your appetite and weight will stabilize, and your metabolism will be able to run at its most efficient.

So, balance = a slimmer, happier you!

Now take pen and paper and write it down:

> *'Balance = a slimmer, happier me!'*

Key Points to Remember
- Since we have been unable to eradicate famine in the world, our body hasn't yet eradicated the natural fast–feast instinct.
- Our body self-regulates food intake through sensory specific satiety and caloric compensation.
- It is frustrating putting all the weight back on when we've just spent several weeks (or months) starving ourselves to lose it, but the body is merely trying to achieve *balance.*
- To beat yo-yo dieting, weight fluctuation, bingeing and simple overeating, *balance* is the key.

- If we eat a varied and balanced diet without restrictions or cravings, as much as the body requires but not to excess, long term, the body will trust that famine is not an issue, and appetite, weight and metabolism will stabilize.
- A 'balanced diet' is considered the healthiest long term, rather than diets which reduce or eliminate entire food groups.

Powerful Food Habit Number Ten

Exercise Snacking Control

Here are 11 simple strategies to use as a checklist to empower you to control snacking and 'grazing'!

1. '*No* more excuses – I don't need this snack!' Write it down! As many times as it takes until the urge goes away.
2. Find another way to get the boost you're looking for and try *that* first, *before* eating!
3. Accept the law of cause and effect: snacking *does* make you fat! So drink water instead, fizzy if you want a little volume – it won't make you fat!
4. If you really must snack, use variety to break the habit. Snack on salty if you like sweet, soft if you like crunchy, and vice versa. Or try postponing the time you usually snack to break the cycle – you might simply be doing it by the clock and once the time has passed, the urge will pass too. Wait 20 minutes at least.
5. Make it a rule to eat only protein as a snack. It'll act as an appetite suppressant and you're less likely to want that snack if it's going to be cheese or ham or a boiled egg instead of biscuits or cake.
6. Write down a couple of healthy snacks you'll allow yourself daily, one mid-morning and one mid-afternoon. Allow yourself no less and no more. Pre-prepare them and have them easy to hand.
7. Before eating the snack, try picking it up and putting it down again. Try putting it down and walking out of the room, or putting it back in the fridge. You're sending signals to your brain that you don't need it…

8. Eat less at mealtimes and allocate part of your meals as a snack. For example, postpone the fruit or yogurt you'd have for dessert so that you can eat it later on. You'll probably enjoy it more that way, too!

9. If you work or are away from home, make a rule that you'll only eat at mealtimes. This not only prevents you buying unnecessary snacks, but also trains your mind to understand that if you're busy, you have no need to snack. It also trains you to feel hungry only at mealtimes. And in addition it can save you a lot of money!

10. If all else fails, keep a bowl of pre-cut 'sweet' veggies at the front and in the lower sections of the fridge right to hand. Red and yellow peppers, sweet cherry tomatoes and cucumber sticks are great options. Blueberries are also very healthy, but stick to a small portion (one small handful), as they contain fructose. If you feel you must snack on something 'non-veg', [11] raw almonds are a high-protein, healthy super-food snack.

11. Only allow yourself to eat carrot sticks as a snack. You'll soon get bored of them and realize that if you were truly hungry you'd eat them anyway, but the feeling of 'Not another carrot stick!' tells you that you aren't really hungry at all! This works wonders with my children. When they try to convince me they want sweets as a snack, I tell them, 'If you're really hungry, you'll have a carrot!'

5

Be Nutritionally Aware and Exercise Savvy

Let's be blunt: modern life is all about convenience and quick and ready solutions – how to do the most with the least effort and time, and sadly sometimes with the least personal commitment or responsibility.

But making sustainable change can never be about a quick fix. There are no 'quick fixes' in transformation! Because to transform your body shape, your health or your life in any way at all, you have to make a commitment: that's right, a commitment! And commitments, as we all know, are not quick fixes. They're long-term fixes.

Sustainable Change

People generally don't like the idea of commitment, but it is what separates the achievers from the non-achievers, the heroes from the zeroes, the super-rich from the average Joe, and, yes, the fat from the slim! Commitment means making a plan and taking action so that you start, progress and finish on the right road to accomplishing that plan. It means putting in the work and the focus and the effort day after day, hour after hour. It means learning from failures as well as successes and tailoring your actions to make sure you do better next time. It means a long-term view and a long-term plan. *Not* a quick fix or a miracle cure.

Anyone who hopes to achieve weight loss through a short-term solution or a miracle cure or a quick fix isn't committed to losing weight. Period. Full stop. Because if you're not willing to put in the long-term commitment, focus and effort, you're doomed to failure.

The motivator and coach Chris Howard puts it like this: 'You have to have skin in the game,' which means that you have to invest *your* own effort in any endeavour you want to succeed in. Just as in business, you have to have a stake in it to win.

And quick fixes in the world of losing weight and getting fitter can never work. This has to do with how our metabolism works and our body lays down fat. By drastically reducing your calorie intake through crash diets or quick fixes, you are actually reducing your body's ability to burn calories in the future. When the body is deprived of fuel, the metabolic rate slows down to compensate (burning energy more slowly so that it lasts longer). Basically, your body is readjusting its fuel consumption in response to a perceived risk of famine.

Crash diets may cause fast weight loss initially, but this is only because your body initially uses up the glycogen (carbohydrate and sugar) stored in the liver and the muscles, as well as the water which is stored with it. The water released accounts for much of the 'weight' lost when you look at the scales. Next is muscle loss, unless the diet is a very high-protein regime. Muscle loss, in particular, slows down the metabolic rate because muscle mass burns up more calories gram for gram than fat, so the more muscle mass you have, the more calories you burn (even at rest), and vice versa. So, guess what? The decrease in muscle mass from crash dieting means a long-term decrease in your ability to burn calories efficiently. What's more, weight will quickly be put back on, as the slower metabolism will be unable to efficiently process an increase in calories once normal eating is resumed. With the excess stored as fat where the now-lost muscle mass used to be, your body is now programmed to burn fewer calories gram for gram of body weight.

Quite apart from this effect on your metabolism, crash diets often lack crucial vitamins and minerals, potentially affecting your skin tone and radiance, the health of your hair and nails, your energy and mood and even your reproductive health and libido!

So even if you were to lose weight on a crash diet, to prevent putting it all back on again you'd have to change your eating habits radically and permanently as well as exercising like mad to increase your muscle mass. Even then the odds are stacked against you. It is unlikely that the weight lost so quickly wouldn't creep back on. Remember that the body has an in-built weight 'barometer' in the hypothalamus, called the ponderostat, which 'defends the preferred body mass'[1] by managing the signals which control our metabolism and feeding behaviour. This means that a rapid decrease in weight will naturally lead to the scales tipping back the other way to redress the body's perceived natural balance. What's more, medical research suggests that 'energy deficit results in heightened taste responsiveness',[2] especially when weight is dropped below the 'set point' regulated by the ponderostat. In layman's terms, this means that when you crash diet, everything may start to taste better to force you to put weight back on again!

Don't forget, too, that crash diets are imbalanced and can lead to binge-eating as compensation, or to yo-yo dieting. The intense deprivation they entail can wreak havoc with our natural self-control and cause unhealthy food obsessions, which are often the basis of eating disorders.

Quoting from a medical journal:

> '...VLCD (Very Low Calorie Diets) are as ineffective as conventional diets when we evaluate them in the long term. This is why traditional weight loss treatments have recently been questioned, in addition to the unsuccessful results, for the psychological costs: eating disorders because of restriction and deprivation, reduction of self-esteem ... body unsatisfaction, irritability, increased anxiety and depression... All this indicates that [it] is necessary [to have] a long-term dietary programme, based on education about food and eating habits ... gradual weight loss preventing negative psychological consequences ... being as flexible as possible to prevent failure.'[3]

Remember that the UK National Health Service recommends the 'slowly and surely' method of losing weight: a safe level of 1–2lb a week (just under half a kilo to a kilogram).

Remember, too, that in any case exercise speeds up the metabolic rate and increases muscle mass, so it should be an integral part of any weight-loss, weight-maintenance or healthy-living plan!

More on exercise, later, but now let's look at 'super-foods'...

'Super-foods'

Some foods are veritable powerhouses of health, vitality and goodness. Nowadays, they are becoming known as 'super-foods'. These foods are especially relevant to the exciting new field of 'Nutrigenomics', as explained by Stephen Pratt, MD, author of the *New York Times* bestseller *SuperFoodsRx*:

> 'Scientists are now discovering that not all of the food we eat is metabolized for energy. A small percentage of dietary chemicals become ligands – molecules that bind to proteins involved in "turning on" certain genes.'[4]

So the foods we eat can turn on or off the genes that are responsible for our state of health! One such 'super-nutrient' found in many super-foods is Resveratrol, a potent antioxidant which can help decrease the risk of heart disease and is found in peanuts, purple and red grapes, blueberries, cranberries and red wine. Super-foods also contain 'phyto-nutrients', which are non-vitamin or non-mineral nutrients with proven health benefits.

Super-foods also play a large part in helping to eliminate and control inflammation in the body. Inflammation is the underlying factor in almost all of our modern diseases and epidemics, including cardiovascular disease, types of cancer, arthritis, Crohn's disease, diabetes, irritable bowel syndrome and even cataracts.

Many super-foods are also good sources of dietary fibre. Dietary fibre lowers the glycaemic index of the food, helping us to fill up more quickly and stay satisfied for longer, and in so doing, helps to control blood sugar levels, reduce stomach fat and keep the bowels and intestine healthy and regular, as well as decreasing the risk of diabetes and atherosclerosis (hardening of the arteries).

Other super-substances found in the various super-foods are (and this is by no means an exhaustive list!):

- antioxidants (the substances that neutralize the 'free radicals' in our body which cause cellular ageing
- essential vitamins
- probiotics (great for gastro-intestinal health and keeping slim)
- enzymes
- flavanoids (found in cocoa, tea, cranberries and other fruits) which protect your skin and have antioxidant properties: tea polyphenol has anti-cancer and anti-inflammatory properties![5]
- polyphenols (*see above*)
- B vitamins and folic acid, which help control atherosclerosis and inflammation

So what are you waiting for? Super-foods are just waiting to help you to be your healthiest and most energetic, slow down and reverse ageing, and protect you from the common diseases of the 21st century, as well as gain a trim physique! You'll find a list of *'Super-foods'* in Appendix II at the back of this book.

The Toxicity Trap

by Erica Jones, CEO of designerhealthcenters.com

Many people might be very surprised to know that the vast majority of food consumed in this day and age isn't really food. Our grocery store aisles are lined with nutrient-depleted, chemically processed, fake foods that most people consume on a daily basis without even a second thought! These foods play a key role in the onset of many diseases, especially our modern overweight and obesity epidemics. Part of the struggle is that many people simply aren't aware that what they are consuming daily can have extremely damaging effects, not only hampering their quality of life (weight problems, fatigue, hormonal imbalance, etc.), but, most dramatically, substantially increasing a risk of chronic disease! Who would consciously choose that?

What you need to be aware of is that food manufacturers have a vested interest in you buying their products to increase their profitability. To do this they need to make sure that their products taste the best they possibly can – even if this is at the expense of the food's underlying nutritional quality! For this reason, many food products have been infused with 'extras' (or what, in my job, I encounter as toxins!) designed to enhance the flavour, shelf life or palatability. Unfortunately, these food 'enhancers' don't enhance our health – instead they can take a serious toll, especially when consumed in excess.

Quite simply, there are three main food 'toxins' that you need to avoid as much as possible: high-fructose corn syrup (HFCS), bad fats and chemical preservatives. These three are so commonly used in food products today that an average person with a conventional diet is consuming them in excess. That's nearly everyone! These substances are not even limited to 'junk' foods like potato chips and soda pop. They have already found their way into foods which are advertised as healthy – which couldn't be further from the truth! This presentation and marketing makes these particular ingredients even more dangerous, because the foods they are concealed in are not obviously 'harmful' in the same way as a bowl of candy!

This is all the more reason why we should – each and every one of us – take the time to educate ourselves and be more diligent about what we are eating. Empowering yourself with education will give you the tools that you need to make healthy choices. And help is at hand! Use *'Powerful Food*

Habit Number One: Read Food Labels' in Chapter 4 of this book, as your primary resource: check if the three food toxins are actually ingredients in foods you'd like to buy or you consume regularly!

High-Fructose Corn Syrup

The old saying is that anything can be consumed in moderation. Well, things have changed a bit in modern times! As Natasha Reddy expertly points out in the *'The Sugar Trap'* (coming up in a few pages' time), high-fructose corn Syrup (HFCS) is one substance to avoid: in fact, I'd urge everyone not to consume it at all – not even in moderation! Why, you might ask, such a strong reaction to a little bit of sugar or corn syrup? Well, in my business of running one of the premier health centre chains in the Americas and the Middle East (guarding people's health from the source rather than simply curing symptoms), it's a little bit more complicated than that!

HFCS use has increased dramatically in use in the past several years. This particular sweetening agent appeals strongly to food manufacturers because it's cheap, maintains a long shelf life and tastes good. For this reason, HFCS has made its way into many pre-packaged foods and snacks you find in your local grocery or convenience store, especially in the US. But these flavour-enhanced products, and their cheap cost, do not come without consequences – and unfortunately mainstream society (people just like you and me) is the one to pay for it.

If you've ever wondered how it's possible to eat a whole tub of ice-cream without a second thought, then wonder no more! Sugary snacks, ice-cream, cookies, pastries, cereals, breakfast bars, frozen dinners and especially soft drinks are often absolutely loaded with HFCS. Research has shown that sugar can override the body's normal signals of satiation, which can (and does) lead to overeating.[6] This is the root cause of addictive behaviour when it comes to food – which is why it can be so darn easy to eat a whole bag of cookies! It's not your fault: it's sugar and its substitutes suppressing the body's ability to recognize the point at which we should feel full and satisfied.

The consequences of this are terrible! Overeating leads to being overweight and obese (especially when sugar is the primary source) and then weight-management issues come with their own list of risk factors, which include heart disease, diabetes, cancer and high cholesterol!

If you want to reduce your intake of HFCS and other sugars, you'll need to make sure that you do read food labels. You should also try your best to avoid or at least reduce your consumption of soft drinks (a primary source of HFCS) and sugary snacks.

Bad Fats

When most people think about bad fats they think of deep-fried foods and trans (or hydrogenated) fats. Many of us know from recent negative publicity that these fats should definitely be avoided, but unfortunately that's only part of the story. In the same way that HFCS has made its way into many products on the grocery aisle, bad fats in the form of vegetable oils are right there alongside!

Excess consumption of vegetable oils can cause a myriad of health issues. Liver damage, decreased immune function, rapid ageing and wrinkles, anyone? (Gasp!) These are just some of the repercussions, along with many other health issues.[7] Some of the most common vegetable oils found in many processed foods are canola oil, soybean oil and cottonseed oil – in addition to your standard 'vegetable oil'. However, many of these may be hydrogenated or partially hydrogenated (trans-fat) oils, which you can be sure won't help you lose weight or increase your overall health and vitality. Natasha tells me that in the UK several major upmarket supermarket chains have taken the initiative to ban hydrogenated fats and oils from their product ranges, which is absolutely great and proof that the dangers of these fats are finally being recognized by the mainstream!

Other bad fats to avoid are butter substitutes, margarine and squeezable butters. These products typically contain vegetable oils *and* partially hydrogenated (trans) fats. Again, the best way to be sure that you're avoiding these harmful foods is to be diligent about reading food labels. You deserve to know what's going into your body!

Chemical Preservatives

We all like the convenience of being able to reach into the cupboard to enjoy a snack when we're walking out the door or when we just don't feel like taking the time to prepare something. Foods allowing us this convenience usually have a long shelf life. Well, the convenience doesn't come without a cost!

In order to maintain that long shelf life, foods need additives called preservatives in order to maintain freshness over time. Unfortunately, most preservatives are chemicals conjured up in a laboratory! To add insult to injury, some commonly used preservatives have been shown to cause cancer in lab animals. For example, BHA (butylated hydroxyanisole) is an antioxidant and waxy solid used as a food additive with the E number E320.[8] BHA and BHT (butylated hydroxytoluene), also known as butylhydroxytoluene, an antioxidant food additive (E number E321) also used in embalming fluid (yikes!)[9] can be found in many breads, cereals, chips, baked goods and other snacks! These two chemicals have been linked to tumours in lab mice! Many other preservatives are similarly questionable.

Though they are not preservatives, food colourings are often added to cereals and snacks, especially those marketed toward children! Some food dyes (Red 3 and Yellow 4 for example) have also been flagged as carcinogenic in tests. But they're still being added to our foods! Sadly, the list goes on and on. There are hundreds, perhaps even thousands more additives and preservatives that haven't even been tested but are no doubt similarly detrimental to our health and still finding their way into our grocery store aisles!

What You Can Do

First, what you *shouldn't* do is get bogged down and overwhelmed. There are so many harmful ingredients and products on the market that to discuss each and every one would be beyond the scope of this book. What you *should* do is exercise diligence to the best of your ability whenever you're eating a meal or snack. Do what you *can* do! Typically, this means that you should choose whole foods as opposed to those full of chemicals, oils or sugar. The reality is that you'll be hard pressed to find packaged food products that contain many (if any) foods without chemicals, preservatives, additives and so on. This is why it's so extremely important to implement *'Powerful Food Habit Number Two: Get Fresh!'* (Chapter 4), which is all about eating fresh, natural food. Infusing your diet with delicious whole foods, fruits and vegetables is a very effective way of losing weight and increasing your energy and your overall health and well-being. By eating more fresh produce, you'll automatically reduce your intake of highly processed toxic foods. Eating whole foods is a major part of our detoxification and weight-loss programmes at Designer Health Centers. And we see the life-changing results in our clients (thousands of them around the world) each and every day!

There's no point in learning new information if you don't take action on what you've learned. We already know that obesity, overweight, cancer, heart disease, diabetes, hypertension and high cholesterol are running rampant in our industrialized nations and other parts of the world. The convenience that we have come to know (and love) from ready-made, pre-packaged, highly processed foods is a major contributing factor to the decline in health in nations all over the world. So, know from now on that these advances in food technology do not come without a cost to our health and our overall quality of life – and act upon this knowledge!

The harmful effects of processed foods and their chemically saturated ingredients are very real. If you choose to do nothing, then you'll be in the same boat as everyone else: at an elevated risk of obesity, cancer, heart disease – the list goes on! You deserve more than that and you owe it to yourself to care! We can't afford to be indifferent about what we eat, because (not to be morbid) the quality of our lives and indeed our lives themselves truly depend on making the right choices. I fully trust that this book will be an invaluable resource to you as from now on you choose health and well-being!

To true health and real results,

Erica Jones

The Sugar Trap

Sugar is universally loved – and for good reason. It increases palatability, which was useful to early man to signal nutritional value as well as to reassure that the food wasn't poisonous (poisonous foods are often bitter). Breast milk is sweet, and sugar-water calms infants more than unsweetened liquid. Sweet fruits were once eaten only in season, their sugar content crucial to build up calorie reserves in summer and autumn before the long lean winter months. Our modern hyper-consumption of sugar, however, was not what nature intended – and has had dire consequences for our health and well-being.

Why You Need to Dump the Sugar

In 2010, US First Lady Michelle Obama launched her 'Let's Move!' campaign to help combat childhood obesity, an affliction affecting around 33 per cent of American children. According to Erica Jones, CEO of designerhealthcenters.com, the average daily consumption of added sugar (meaning sugar not naturally present in foods, being either added during manufacture, processing or at table) currently stands at a whopping 22.2 teaspoons per adult, and 14 to 18 is 34.3 teaspoons per day per child.

People who eat a diet rich in sugar tend to be overweight, whether the sugar source is sucrose (table sugar), high-fructose corn syrup (HFCS), fructose, or the sugar-rich marinades, salad dressings, soups, pasta sauces (even cold sliced meats injected with sugar syrup) which are increasingly making their way onto our dining tables, sneaking in gram after gram of hidden sugar – not half as obvious as a doughnut covered in icing, but just as deadly!

In fact, sugar produces surges of dopamine, the 'feel-good' hormone, in the brain centre linked to pleasure, the *nucleus accumbens*. The same surges occur after the consumption of opiate drugs – better known as morphine and opium – as well as amphetamines and cocaine. This alarming fact should be enough to convince anyone that sugar is literally addictive – and, in excess, dangerous.

In his fascinating book *The End of Overeating*, Dr David Kessler states:

> 'Foods high in sugar, fat, and salt, and the cues that signal them, promote more of everything: more arousal … more thoughts of food … more urge to pursue food … more dopamine-stimulated approach behaviour … more consumption … more opioid-driven reward … more overeating to feel better … more delay in feeling full … more loss of control … more preoccupation with food … more habit-driven behaviour … and ultimately, more and more weight gain … Hyperpalatable foods are hyperstimulants. And when a stimulant produces reward, we want more of it … the reward circuits targeted by highly palatable food are also the reward circuits targeted by drugs.'[10]

It is sugar that makes food taste good and, according to Dr Kessler, when sugar is combined with fat and salt in the right quantities (the very lucrative 'recipe' of fast and processed foods) the 'hyperpalatability' that results is one of the main causes of 21st-century obesity.

But being overweight is not the only symptom of a sugar-rich diet. So are modern epidemics such as diabetes – especially Type 2, otherwise known as 'late onset' diabetes.[11] Diabetes is not only on the rise in the Coca-Cola-guzzling and doughnut-munching Western world: India, China and south-east Asia are following suit as their consumption of refined sugar rises. And diabetes is particularly insidious where Western sugar-loaded drinks, snacks and meals are added to the staple diet based on refined white rice (as in India, China and south-east Asia), because refined rice in itself is a high-GI food.

As well as diabetes, obesity is also linked to hypertension (high blood pressure) and heart disease. And hypertension and diabetes further contribute to kidney disorders and kidney disease.

Lastly, we have metabolic syndrome. This is not exactly a disease in itself, but more a collection of 'markers', including abdominal obesity, elevated triglycerides (blood fats), low 'good' (HDL) cholesterol, high fasting blood glucose levels and high blood pressure, which indicate a risk factor for most – if not all – of the diseases I mentioned above.

According to Dr Richard J. Johnson in his powerful book *The Sugar Fix*, having metabolic syndrome 'doubles your odds of suffering a heart attack and increases by fivefold your chances of developing Type 2 diabetes. Clearly, it is in your interest to avoid developing metabolic syndrome – and your smartest step towards that goal is to consume less fructose.'[12]

Now, you may have noticed that Dr Johnson talks about 'fructose' rather than 'sugar'. What's the difference? Isn't it supposed to be sucrose – 'table' sugar – that's the enemy?

In fact, 'table' sugar is composed of half sucrose and half fructose, one molecule of each, so it's called a 'disaccharide'. We know fructose as fruit sugar, but it's also in honey (about 70 per cent) and in vegetables (in small amounts) – and in the processed sweetener high-fructose corn syrup (HFCS), which is used increasingly as a sweetener, in the US in particular, especially in soft drinks and other processed foods. Fructose is a monosaccharide – the simplest form of sugar which cannot be broken down further (as is glucose). All sugars provide four calories per gram, but some are sweeter than others, fructose being the sweetest, sucrose two thirds as sweet and glucose about half as sweet. Lactose and galactose, the natural sugars present in milk, are, luckily, the only sugars you really don't have to worry about, because of the benefits of the calcium in milk: calcium aids the body in burning fat and regulating blood pressure.

While eating too much of any type of sugar will cause weight gain, fructose deserves a special mention for being particularly problematic. Dr Johnson and other researchers have discovered that a fructose-rich diet in particular not only causes rapid weight gain but, more worrying in the long term, does not appear to satisfy the appetite, so sabotaging weight loss. This is because high-fructose foods may interfere with the neurological signalling process that tells the brain that we are full (why this is the case will be explained later).

This is especially worrying because fructose constitutes an increasingly large part of our modern diet. HFCS, for example, is cheaper than 'table' sugar and used to sweeten a large array of soft drinks, ketchups, sauces, crackers and snacks – even soups. Beware especially of fruit 'juices' labelled 'drink', 'cocktail' or 'punch', or anything except 'juice', which means that they aren't pure juice and are sweetened instead by large amounts of sugar or HFCS. Soft drinks are just like a syringe delivering fructose and sugar directly into the bloodstream. So people who drink a lot of fruit juice and sweetened drinks put on weight easily and quickly!

Fructose is broken down in the liver by an enzyme called 'fructokinase' and transformed into either glycogen (the way sugar is stored in the muscle) or triglycerides (the form in which fat is stored in our cells). Research at the University of California at Davis has also shown that high levels of fructose cause high triglyceride levels (linked to diabetes and cardiovascular disease) as well as below-normal levels of HDL (the good cholesterol which offers protection against cardiovascular disease.)[13]

Some studies have even shown that high-fructose diets cause insulin resistance (where cells cannot use insulin effectively – the precursor to metabolic syndrome and Type 2 diabetes).[14] Insulin, you will remember, is the hormone released by the pancreas in response to blood sugar levels rising and its job is to 'escort' sugar into the cells in order to store it in the form of glycogen, at which point blood sugar levels drop. For a long time fructose has been an ally to diabetics, because it triggers the release of only moderate amounts of insulin. For this reason it has a reasonably low GI rating, but must be treated nevertheless with great caution.

However, insulin also triggers the release of leptin, the 'feel full' hormone, which acts on the brain to induce satiety, triggers the decrease of grehlin, the hunger-producing hormone, helps to increase the metabolic rate and regulates triglyceride storage. But because fructose only triggers moderate amounts of insulin, it also has 'little or no effect on appetite hormones', according to Dr. Johnson and studies at the University of California at Davis.[15] In effect, fructose doesn't stimulate leptin production – or the mechanism that tells you you're full. This means that after eating fructose-rich foods your appetite may not be satisfied, making you consume more and, of course, store more in the form of fat! What's worse, this 'shutting-off' of the appetite hormone may eventually occur for all types of food, even those which don't actually contain fructose, if the body has been subjected to it on a consistent basis...

In conclusion, whatever our gender, weight, age and lifestyle, reducing our intake of all types of sugars is an indisputably positive step to not only a slimmer physique, but, most importantly, to better health. The modest amounts of natural sugars in our diet from eating no more than a couple of pieces of fruit per day, as well as vegetables, should be sufficient. There's no excuse for consuming hidden, processed and added sugars in any shape or form. Learn to read labels to root out these hidden dangers to our health! After my father had a heart-valve replacement operation, my mother was quick to start making all her own pasta sauces and salad dressings – all without sugar of course, but just as tasty, if not much tastier, than the sugar-rich commercial versions!

Just to underline to you sugars included in processed foods, here's the ingredient list for a bag of 'freshly-baked home-style' American-style cookies from an upmarket food store – and quite expensive at that. I have put all the different types of sugar in italics (including whey powder, which is a source of lactose, milk sugar):

> 'Wheat flour, *sugar*, butter, white Belgian chocolate chunks (*sugar*, *milk powder*, cocoa butter, emulsifier soya lecithin, flavouring), dried cranberries (*sugar*, cranberries, sunflower oil), water, *dextrose monohydrate*, *sucrose*, *fructose*, wheat fibre, *lactose*, raising agents calcium phosphates, disodium diphosphate and sodium hydrogen carbonate, *vegetarian whey powder*, *black treacle*, *maltose*, salt, flavouring.'

There are 11 sugar sources listed in just one cookie – how scary is that? Of the remaining ingredients, refined wheat flour converts rapidly to blood sugar, butter, cocoa butter and sunflower oil are all fats, and all that's left is (token) wheat fibre, a few token cranberries, water, salt and flavouring and a few raising agents which sound as though they belong in the laboratory. I don't know about you, but there's no way I'm giving these to my children!

What about Sweeteners?

What are generally referred to as 'artificial sweeteners' are many times sweeter than sugar, bestow few or no calories and have little effect on blood sugar levels. So far, so good. But we all know that many artificial sweeteners are dogged by controversy. So, what's the problem?

Well, the word 'artificial', for starters, for those which really are. Not all sweeteners are artificial – some are derived from natural products.

Here are some of the commonly-used sweeteners on the market today:

- xylitol, sorbitol, mannitol, maltitol, lactitol, isolmalt and glycerol, referred to as 'polyols'
- saccharin ('Sweet'n'Low' in pink packets)
- sucralose ('Splenda')
- aspartame ('Nutrasweet', 'Canderel' and 'Equal')
- acelsufame-K ('Sweet One')
- Stevia

The polyols, also known as 'sugar alcohols', despite containing neither substance, are derived from natural products. Not being as sweet as sucrose, they are often used in conjunction with high-intensity artificial sweeteners to combat the latter's slightly bitter aftertaste. Being incompletely absorbed into the bloodstream and metabolized, they have a limited (but not negligible) effect on blood sugar, which makes them attractive to diabetics and those on low-carbohydrate diets. However, for this very same reason, they can produce flatulence and diarrhoea if consumed in large quantities.

Nevertheless, unlike artificial sweeteners, sugar alcohols are *not* calorie-free and have been known to stall weight loss, especially if consumed regularly or in quantity, because, as mentioned above, their effect on blood sugar isn't negligible (and in excess can be comparable to fructose), so their use has to be controlled by diabetics and those on a weight-loss plan.[16]

Saccharin (also known as the food additive E954) is the oldest of all artificial sweeteners, having been discovered in 1878 at John Hopkins University. After widespread controversy following the development of bladder cancer in rats fed with saccharin, it was found that this side-effect could not be translated to humans due to biological differences, and in December 2010 the US Environmental Protection Agency finally removed it from its Hazardous Substances Listing. The FDA no longer considers it any threat to human health. However, although it has no calories, apparently it can trigger the release of insulin due to its sweet taste and is best avoided in favour of other sweeteners.[17]

Sucralose, or 'Splenda', was (ironically) discovered by scientists from the British Tate & Lyle sugar company. It contains no calories, doesn't cause dental cavities, doesn't affect insulin levels and has been registered as safe for human consumption by various international food regulatory bodies. Aspartame (food additive E951), on the other hand, has developed a bad name, mainly because of many concerns as to its safety, none of which has been conclusively proven. Nevertheless, it should not be consumed in pregnancy or by people with a rare genetic condition called phenylketonuria (wherein aspartame becomes toxic when metabolized). It has been stated that 'the weight of existing scientific evidence indicates that aspartame is safe at current levels of consumption as a non-nutritive sweetener'.[18] However, aspartame has also been shown to trigger the release of insulin due to its sweet taste, in the same way as saccharin.[19]

Acelsufame-K (food additive E950) is as sweet as aspartame and is almost always used in conjunction with it or another sweetener, such as sucralose. Although FDA approved for general use, critics note it may be carcinogenic and advocate further studies, although these claims are disputed by regulatory authorities.

Lastly, Stevia deserves a special mention. It is a species of chrysanthemum-like tropical and sub-tropical shrub which is native to South America. Its derivative steviol glycoside is hundreds of times sweeter than sugar and has negligible effect on blood sugar. It has allegedly been used for centuries to sweeten the South American drink *mate* and as a treatment for diabetes, and has been used as a sweetener in Japan (in diet Coca-Cola), Korea and China for decades. Despite an earlier ban by the FDA (based on inadequate information to determine its safety) it is now allowed as a dietary supplement (or 'herb') in the United States, but not as a food additive. At the time of writing, it had yet to be approved by Hong Kong or Singapore, but was already appearing on the shelves in the U.K and Canada: it is certainly a sweetener worth considering! It responds well to cooking, being heat-stable (despite not adding bulk), is non-calorific, does not raise insulin levels, allegedly contains medicinal properties and is easily cultivated.

The Benefits of PHA Exercise

Right, now back to exercise! We all know about the benefits of exercise, but sadly we don't all enjoy those benefits! Thing is, exercise has to be easy, fun and quick, or we won't make the effort. But when it *is* easy, fun and quick, it doesn't feel like effort at all!

How would you like to boost your metabolism and burn body fat to gain a leaner, firmer and more balanced body in just 20 minutes, three or four times a week, without spending hours on the treadmill or at the gym?

Peripheral Heart Action (PHA) training was developed by Dr Arthur Steinhaus and then popularized by Bob Gajda – 'Mr America' in 1966! Allegedly Bruce Lee, the martial arts legend, also followed a PHA training programme. The PHA system is designed to keep blood circulating throughout the whole body during exercise. To do this it alternates between upper and lower body exercises interspersed with short bursts of aerobic activity, giving your heart and lungs a real workout as they maintain constant blood and oxygen flow. And because you're not 'exerting' yourself in the old-fashioned sense of needing a lot of stamina, you're avoiding feeling that it's too much effort, because you're constantly changing the variety of movement. This also helps to prevent muscle fatigue – you should never get as far as feeling that muscle 'burn'!

What's so good about PHA is that it maximizes the results from your effort in a very short period of time, but still increases cardiovascular (heart and lungs) fitness, strength and fat-burning! It also raises your basal metabolic rate, the rate at which your body burns food for energy and maintenance even when at rest.

What's more, PHA training can be done anywhere! Once you are familiar with some basic exercises, you can do them at the gym, park or your own home, using household objects and skipping ropes instead of gym machines and weights. And it doesn't matter what your level of fitness is, because with the wide variety of exercises within a short timescale you can tailor it to your own requirements and you needn't get bored either!

So why do I advocate PHA exercise rather than just a simple jog or a few lengths of the pool? Quite simply because it's most suited to fat-burning and muscle-toning, which is what people want most of all!

Here's the layout of a simple PHA workout, called a 'cycle':[20]

1. Compound leg exercise, like a simple lunge.

2. Upper body pushing exercise, like the chest press in the gym or using cans of food at home!
3. Compound leg exercise, like squats.
4. Upper body pulling exercise, like 'lat pull-downs' at the gym.
5. 'Cardio' (like jogging or 'Step' or Cycle, where you exercise heart and lungs).

All exercises in the cycle are repeated 10–12 or 15–20 times, and then the cycle is repeated 3–5 times over. Rest as little as possible between each exercise, but enjoy a few minutes' pause between each cycle.

If you want to make the workout more powerful, five-minute bursts of cardio activity (like a five-minute sprint on the treadmill or five minutes of skipping) before your pause and between each cycle will do the trick!

Do you see now why I think PHA exercise is a winner? I mean, only five-minute bursts of exercise at any one time? That's really not that much work, is it, in exchange for real fat-burning, a lean and fit body, and great health?

Rest assured that this type of routine is definitely very accessible to anyone, whatever your weight or shape. You can start gently and tailor the different exercises to your own needs. If you're overweight and do a PHA routine three times a week under the guidance of a trainer at the gym, you are guaranteed to burn fat and lean up without over-exertion. You'll even have fun, because the variations are endless – there's no time to get bored or even to feel like complaining!

The best book on the market in my opinion is Matt Roberts' *The PHA Workout*, so if you want to learn more about this very effective exercise method, check it out.

6

The 28-Day Food Awareness Plan

This plan is specially designed to increase your awareness of how your body reacts to the different food groups. It will definitely help you to eat more mindfully by focusing your awareness on your reactions to various foods. As a side-effect, it may help you to lose excess weight, gain energy and combat weight-loss resistance! Once you are aware of how you and your body behave with regards to the different food groups, and how these make you feel, you will have gained greater control over your diet, your appetite, your weight and your health.

This plan is designed to be used in combination with the rest of this book. The most important thing is to take it slowly and concentrate on tasting the food properly. It is also advisable to note down your feelings before and after your food. Compiling a daily journal is an important part of this process (*'Powerful Food Habit Number Six'* in Chapter 4 of this book will guide you).

Ideally, this plan should be optimally combined with an exercise routine (*'The Benefits of PHA Exercise'* at the end of Chapter 5, you've just read it!).

How does the plan work? It uniquely rotates different combinations of healthy 'regimes' within a short-term framework, so that they are optimized in a productive, benign way and cross-interact for maximum efficiency. It is designed to kick-start the metabolism and turn off the bodily mechanisms which cause weight-loss resistance. Its 'zig-zag' approach combats boredom as well as allowing individual freedom to plan menus – in a word, it's *sustainable*! It rotates between pure lean protein, lean protein plus low-

GI vegetables, adds in medium-GI fruit and vegetables, and finally adds in healthy low-GI grains and carbohydrates. This incremental pattern is designed to prevent cravings or feelings of deprivation. (At the end of this chapter you'll find full lists of the foods allowed under the various categories; see *'Food Lists'*.)

The plan lasts 28 days for those with less than 10lb to lose, or doubles up as an eight-week plan for those with 10lb or more to lose. There are three initial phases (Plans A–C), then a transition phase, (Plan D), followed by a maintenance phase (Plan E) and a lifestyle plan (Plan F), as follows:

- *Plan A: 'Shock Start the Metabolism'*: This phase is guaranteed to help speed up your metabolism by giving your body access to lean protein-rich foods whilst eliminating the sugars and carbohydrates that are easily turned into glycogen (blood sugar). There are also no complex carbohydrates for the moment, to avoid the effects of yeast and gas on the body. However, by the end of the week healthy low-GI berries and fruits are introduced.

- *Plan B: 'Train the Metabolism'*: This phase is rather like a more condensed version of Plan A, but further adds in higher-GI fruits at the end of the week to prevent cravings. Complex carbohydrates are still not being introduced while the body is eliminating toxins and water retention.

- *Plan C: 'Reassure the Metabolism'*: This phase, adding the different food groups day by day, finally includes a moderate number of low-GI carbohydrate-rich foods, grains and cereals at the end of the week as well as a small number of starchy vegetables. By now you should be aware of how you feel and react to each of the food groups in turn.

- *Plan D: 'Transition Plan'*: This phase represents the journey back to an everyday balanced and varied diet. It lasts for two weeks, regardless of weight. It is based on the framework of Plan C, but broadens the protein groups by adding in fatty fish high in the omega oils, lean lamb, duck, goose, etc. It also adds small servings of unsalted and raw nuts, dried fruits, one serving of unprocessed cheese and a serving of full-fat yogurt every day. It also includes a 'free meal'.

- *Plan E: 'Maintenance Plan'*: This phase advises sustaining the good dietary and lifestyle lessons you've learned!

Fun Rules

There are a few 'fun rules' to abide by to make sure you're optimizing the plan. Here they are:

1. Do not eat any chemically saturated processed foods for the duration of the plan (in fact you should avoid these inflammation- and disease-producing ageing 'foods' in any case from now on). Only buy and consume 100 per cent fresh and 100 per cent natural/unadulterated foods (the way nature intended), organic if your purse allows it!

2. Limit the use of salt and use all varieties of fresh herbs and natural seasonings instead.

3. Do not consume sugar (sucrose) or foods containing unprocessed sucrose, and limit high-fructose foods for the meantime. This is to aid 'turning off' fructose 'receptors' which may be contributing to your weight-loss resistance. Check all ingredients for hidden sugars – all the 'oses'!

4. Eliminate white and processed carbohydrates for the duration of the plan (you should avoid these in any case from now on, fewer of these equals less weight and more health). These can be tasted occasionally during maintenance, if you choose. Learn about glycaemic index ratings and respect them (read *'Powerful Food Habit Number Four: Do Low GI'* in Chapter 4).

5. Choose your foods from the *'Food Lists'* specified at the end of this section, and stick religiously to these lists for the duration of the plan.

6. No alcohol, unless specified, and no fruit juice. These can be drunk in moderation (the juice in diluted form) during maintenance, if you choose. Drink at least 1.5 litres of filtered or low-sodium mineral water per day throughout the day.

7. Enjoy following the Keys in this book, including *how* to eat, not just *what* to eat!

8. Take exercise – a minimum of half an hour's brisk walk a day. Remember that with exercise you get out what you put in, so more exercise means you'll be healthier, slimmer and fitter! You can find out more in *'The Benefits of PHA Exercise'* at the end of Chapter 5 (the previous Chapter).

9. Keep a journal to track your progress (*'Powerful Food Habit Number Six: Keep a Food Journal'*, in Chapter 4) and don't forget to note down your thoughts and feelings daily.

10. Respect yourself and your health through the choices you make, ensure you get enough sleep, and, most importantly, *fall in love with the process!*

Plan A

'Shock Start' the Metabolism

Duration
Weeks 1 & 2 for up to 10lb overweight.
Weeks 1, 2, 3 & 4 for more than 10lb overweight.

Days 1 and 2

(PP) = *Pure protein* to kick-start the metabolism. This is high-value dense-nutritional-quality *lean* protein cooked without fats. (For recipe ideas, see *'Sample Recipes for the Whole Family'* at the end of this section, after *'Food Lists'*.)

- Nothing else.
- 2 litres of low-sodium mineral water throughout the day in small sips.
- *No* alcohol, tea or coffee except herbal teas and decaffeinated coffee, without milk, if absolutely necessary.

Day 3 and 4

(PP) + (G) = low-GI green super-food vegetables

- *Pure protein* as before.
- Plus low-GI *green* super-food vegetables *only* – no medium-GI coloured vegetables or high-GI starchy vegetables.
- *No* fruit.
- *No* carbohydrate-rich foods or grains or cereals.
- 2 litres of low-sodium mineral water throughout the day in small sips.
- *No* alcohol, tea or coffee except herbal teas and decaffeinated coffee, without milk, if absolutely necessary.

Days 5 and 6

(PP) + (G) + (C) = medium-GI *coloured* super-food vegetables and salads

- *Pure protein* as before.
- Plus low-GI *green* vegetables as before.

- Plus (C) = medium-GI *coloured* super-food vegetables and salads.
- *No* high-GI starchy vegetables.
- *No* fruit.
- *No* carbohydrate-rich foods or grains or cereals.
- 2 litres of low-sodium mineral water throughout the day in small sips.
- *No* alcohol, tea or coffee except herbal teas and decaffeinated coffee, without milk, if absolutely necessary.

Day 7

(PP) + (G) + (C) + (F1) = low-GI *fruit*, max 2 servings of 100g each
- *Pure protein* as before.
- Plus low-GI *green* vegetables as before.
- Plus medium-GI *coloured* super-food vegetables and salads as before.
- Plus (F1) = low-GI *fruit*, max. 2 servings of 100g each.
- *No* high-GI fruit.
- *No* high-GI starchy vegetables.
- *No* carbohydrate-rich foods or grains or cereals.
- 2 litres of low-sodium mineral water throughout the day in small sips.
- *No* alcohol, tea or coffee except herbal teas and decaffeinated coffee, without milk, if absolutely necessary.

Plan B

Train the Metabolism

Duration
Week 3 for up to 10lb overweight.
Weeks 5 & 6 for more than 10lb overweight.

Day 1

(PP) = *Pure protein* to kick-start the metabolism. This is high-value dense-nutritional-quality *lean* protein cooked without fats.

- Nothing else.
- 2 litres of low-sodium mineral water throughout the day in small sips.
- *No* alcohol, tea or coffee except herbal teas and decaffeinated coffee, without milk, if absolutely necessary.

Day 2

(PP) + (G) = low-GI *green* super-food vegetables
- *Pure protein* as before.
- Plus (G) = low-GI *green* super-food vegetables.
- *No* medium-GI *coloured* vegetables or fruit.
- *No* high-GI starchy vegetables.
- *No* fruit.
- *No* carbohydrate-rich foods or grains or cereals.
- 2 litres of low-sodium mineral water throughout the day in small sips.
- *No* alcohol, tea or coffee except herbal teas and decaffeinated coffee, without milk, if absolutely necessary.

Days 3 and 4

(PP) + (G) + (C) = medium-GI *coloured* super-food vegetables and salads
- *Pure protein* as before.
- Plus low-GI *green* vegetables as before.

- Plus (C) = medium-GI *coloured* super-food vegetables and salads.
- *No* high-GI starchy vegetables.
- *No* fruit.
- *No* carbohydrate-rich foods or grains or cereals.
- 2 litres of low-sodium mineral water throughout the day in small sips.
- *No* alcohol, tea or coffee except herbal teas and decaffeinated coffee, without milk, if absolutely necessary.

Days 5 and 6

(PP) + (G) + (C) + (F1) = low-GI *fruit*, max. 2 x 100g servings
- *Pure protein* as before.
- Plus low-GI *green* vegetables as before.
- Plus medium-GI *coloured* super-food vegetables and salads as before.
- Plus (F1) = low-GI *fruit*, max 2 servings of 100g each.
- *No* high-GI fruit.
- *No* high-GI starchy vegetables.
- *No* carbohydrate-rich foods or grains or cereals.
- 2 litres of low-sodium mineral water throughout the day in small sips.
- *No* alcohol, tea or coffee except herbal teas and decaffeinated coffee, without milk, if absolutely necessary.

Day 7

(PP) + (G) + (C) + (F1) + (F2) = high-GI fruit, max. 1 serving of 100g.
- *Pure protein* as before.
- Plus low-GI *green* vegetables as before.
- Plus medium-GI *coloured* super-food vegetables and salads as before.
- Plus low-GI fruit, max 1 serving of 100g, plus (F2) = high-GI fruit max. 1 serving of 100g.
- *No* high-GI starchy vegetables.
- *No* carbohydrate-rich foods or grains or cereals.
- 2 litres of low-sodium mineral water throughout the day in small sips.
- *No* alcohol, tea or coffee except herbal teas and decaffeinated coffee, without milk, if absolutely necessary.

Plan C

Reassure the Metabolism

Duration
Week 4 for up to 10lb overweight.
Weeks 7 & 8 for more than 10lb overweight.

Day 1

(PP) + (G) = low-GI *green* super-food vegetables
- *Pure protein* as before.
- Plus (G) = low-GI *green* super-food vegetables.
- *No* medium-GI *coloured* vegetables or fruit.
- *No* high-GI starchy vegetables.
- *No* fruit.
- *No* carbohydrate-rich foods or grains or cereals.
- 2 litres of low-sodium mineral water throughout the day in small sips.
- *No* alcohol, tea or coffee except herbal teas and decaffeinated coffee, without milk, if absolutely necessary.

Day 2

(PP) + (G) + (C) = medium-GI *coloured* super-food vegetables and salads.
- *Pure protein* as before.
- Plus low-GI *green* vegetables as before.
- Plus (C) = medium-GI *coloured* super-food vegetables and salads.
- *No* high-GI starchy vegetables.
- *No* fruit.
- *No* carbohydrate-rich foods or grains or cereals.
- 2 litres of low-sodium mineral water throughout the day in small sips.
- *No* alcohol, tea or coffee except herbal teas and decaffeinated coffee, without milk, if absolutely necessary.

Day 3

(PP) + (G) + (C) + (F1) = low-GI *fruit*, max. 2 x 100g servings.
- *Pure protein* as before.
- Plus low-GI *green* vegetables as before.
- Plus medium-GI *coloured* super-food vegetables and salads as before.
- Plus (F1) = low-GI *fruit*, max. 2 servings of 100g each.
- *No* high-GI fruit.
- *No* high-GI starchy vegetables.
- *No* carbohydrate-rich foods or grains or cereals.
- 2 litres of low-sodium mineral water throughout the day in small sips.
- *No* alcohol, tea or coffee except herbal teas and decaffeinated coffee, without milk, if absolutely necessary.

Day 4

(PP) + (G) + (C) + (F1) + (F2) = high-GI *fruit*, max 1 serving of 100g.
- *Pure protein* as before.
- Plus low-GI *green* vegetables as before.
- Plus medium-GI *coloured* super-food vegetables and salads as before.
- Plus low-GI *fruit* as before, max. 1 serving of 100g.
- Plus (F2) = high-GI *fruit*, max. 1 serving of 100g.
- *No* high-GI starchy vegetables.
- *No* carbohydrate-rich foods or grains or cereals.
- 2 litres of low-sodium mineral water throughout the day in small sips.
- *No* alcohol, tea or coffee except herbal teas and decaffeinated coffee, without milk, if absolutely necessary.

Days 5 & 6

(PP) + (G) + (C) + (F1) + (F2) + (LG) = *low-GI* carbohydrate-rich foods, grains, cereals, max. 1 serving of 100g.
- *Pure protein* as before.
- Plus low-GI *green* vegetables as before.

- Plus medium-GI *coloured* super-food vegetables and salads as before.
- Plus low-GI *fruit*, max. 1 serving of 100g, plus high-GI fruit as before, max. 1 serving of 100g.
- *No* high-GI starchy vegetables.
- Yes! (LG) = *low-GI* carbohydrate-rich foods, grains, cereals, max. 1 serving of 100g.
- 2 litres of low-sodium mineral water throughout the day in small sips.
- *No* alcohol, tea or coffee except herbal teas and decaffeinated coffee, without milk, if absolutely necessary.

Day 7

(PP) + (G) + (C) + (F1) + (F2) + (LG) + (S) = high-GI starchy vegetables, max. 1 serving of 50g.

- *Pure protein* as before.
- Plus low-GI *green* vegetables, as before.
- Plus medium-GI *coloured* super-food vegetables and salads, as before.
- Plus low-GI *fruit*, max. 1 serving of 100g.
- Plus high-GI fruit, max. 1 serving of 100g.
- Plus *low-GI* carbohydrate-rich foods, grains, cereals, max. 1 serving of 100g.
- Plus (S) = high-GI starchy vegetables, max. 1 serving of 50g.
- 2 litres of low-sodium mineral water throughout the day in small sips.
- *No* alcohol, tea or coffee except herbal teas and decaffeinated coffee, without milk, if absolutely necessary.
- One small added 'treat' of choice of max. 30g weight.

Plan D

Transition Plan

Duration

2 weeks

Repeat Plan C, adding the following protein groups, if liked:

- Healthy but fattier protein such as fatty fish high in omegas, lean lamb, duck and goose, etc. (refer to list).
- Unsalted and raw nuts and unsweetened dried fruits (max. 30g per day for women and 50g for men).
- One serving (40g max.) of cheese, unprocessed.
- One serving of full-fat yogurt with natural fruit.

One 'free meal' is included this week, but only starter and main or starter and dessert are allowed. Instead of dessert one glass of wine may be drunk.

Plan E

Maintenance Plan

Duration

Forever!

- Follow the *Keys*, *Super-Strategies* and *Powerful Food Habits* in this book.
- Eat super-foods (you will find more information and a list of *'Super-foods'* in Appendix II at the back of this book).
- Eat natural, eat fresh, eat unelaborated food.
- Eat (PP) + (G) + (C) + (F1) + (F2) + (LG) most of the time and (PP) + (G) +(C) + (F1) + (F2) + (LG) + (S) only some of the time.
- Revert to Plan A when weight needs to be lost, followed by Plan B and Plan C.
- Basically, eat lean protein, low GI, minimum glucose/artificial additives.
- But of course anything can be 'tasted', as there is nothing off-bounds! Keep quantities small – *three bites* are enough to taste something very fattening or 'less health-conscious'.
- Exercise regularly.
- If you slip up, recalibrate to stay at your 'happy weight'!

Food Lists

These lists are designed to offer a wide range of natural foods to include in the *'28-Day Food Awareness Plan'*. I cannot guarantee that they are fully comprehensive across cultures and countries. However, if you find a favourite exotic fruit or vegetable, meat, grain or type of seafood that has not been included, as long as it is fresh and unprocessed, by all means do include it if you wish – but please do check the glycaemic rating and/or fat content first if you are unsure (easily done nowadays on the internet, or by using one of the many useful books available to buy). You can also cross-reference to the list of *'Super-foods'* in Appendix II at the back of this book.

Pure Protein Foods (PP)

150g portion
all shellfish and shrimp, excluding processed seafood sticks and scampi tails
Atlantic wild salmon
eggs (except duck eggs, which are higher in fat)
farmed trout
free-range organic duck breast, with the fat trimmed off, cooked without skin (cover it with foil to keep it moist and baste with vegetable stock if necessary: the fat is all under the skin with ducks and geese)
free-range organic turkey, chicken and other poultry, without the skin, although it can be cooked with the skin on to keep it moist; the skin may only be eaten if completely cooked and drained of its fat, on the breast, for example, when cooked to very dark brown and parchment-like; beware of pre-prepared or pre-cooked poultry (which very often has added brown sugar to 'brown' the meat, and may even be injected with sugar syrup)
lean organic beef (best free-range and grass-fed), not ribs or rib-eye steak – grilled or roasted without added fats or oils
lean organic veal, grilled or roasted without added fats or oils
low-fat natural cheese (without additives and colourings)
non-fat and non-sweetened cottage cheese, quark, yogurt and milk, preferably organic
soya yogurt and milk (non-sweetened): watch the quantities, because it is higher in fat than standard milk products; preferably fortified with calcium

sustainably-produced fish (if possible), except fresh wild tuna and swordfish (which can contain traces of mercury) – not in breadcrumbs or dusted with flour
tofu (soya 'cheese')

Low-GI *Green* Super-food Vegetables (G)

These can be eaten freely.

artichokes
asparagus
aubergine (eggplant), cooked without fat
bamboo shoots
beansprouts
beans: green, runner, and French
bok choi
broccoli and broccoli sprouts of all types
Brussels sprouts
cabbage
cauliflower
celery
chicory
chives
collard greens
courgettes (zucchini)
cucumbers
edamame (green soya beans)
fennel
French beans
garlic
green peppers (capsicum)
kale
kohrabi
leeks
mushrooms (shiitake variety, though expensive, are rich in iron)
okra (ladies' fingers), cooked without fats or oil
onions
purslane
radicchio

radishes
romaine lettuce
salad leaves of all types
seaweed
shallots/scallions
spinach
spring onions
squash (winter squash)
string beans
Swiss chard
tomatoes (up to two a day)
turnips
watercress

Medium-GI *Coloured* Super-food Vegetables and Salads (C)

80g portion
beetroot
carrots
coloured peppers (capsicum) yellow, orange and red
mange-tout
peas
petit pois
red cabbage
sugar-snap peas
tomatoes (more than two a day)

Low-GI Fruit (F1)

one medium fruit or one handful
apples
berries (fresh, no sugar or syrup or oils added): raspberries, blackberries, strawberries, loganberries, blueberries, (unsweetened) cranberries, boysenberries, fresh blackcurrants, gooseberries, etc.
clementines
grapefruit (white and pink)
guava (fresh)
lemons
limes
Mandarin oranges
plums

rhubarb

Medium to High-GI *Fruit* (F2)

one medium fruit or one handful
apricots
avocados (included in this list not because they are high GI but because they are exceptionally high in good fats)
bananas
cherries
dates
dried apricots (choose the black unsulphured version with no sugar added, often sold as organic)
dried berries with no sugar, fructose or sugar-syrup added
figs
goji berries
grapes
kiwi fruit
lychees (fresh)
mangoes
melon (two medium slices)
nectarines
oranges
papayas
passionfruit
peaches
pears
persimmons
pineapples
pomegranates
prunes
raisins
satsumas
watermelons

*Low-G*I Carbohydrate-rich Foods, Grains, Cereals (LG)

dried weight 80g or cooked weight 100g
amaranth
barley

brown, wild, camargue red and basmati brown rice
buckwheat
Bulgar wheat
chick peas
cous-cous
durum wheat
ground flaxseed
kidney beans
lentils and dhal
millet
oat bran
oats and oatmeal
pasta (durum wheat not egg-pasta)
pearl barley
quinoa (excellent for its protein content)
rye
spelt (especially good for it being alkaline)
split peas
triticale (rye and wheat)
wheat germ

High-GI *Starchy* Vegetables and Grains (S)

80g portion
broad beans
butternut squash
cassava
corn and sweetcorn and polenta (a maize flour/cornmeal derivative)
potatoes (new and 'old')
pumpkins
rice – white, arborio, risotto, pilau, short-grain, parboiled brown (choose brown
or basmati or basmati brown or wild or camargue instead, which are lower GI)
swede
sweet potatoes
turnips

Extra Protein Foods for Plan D (Transition Plan)

100g portion
fatty fish: salmon, sardines, mackerel, scampi
lean lamb
pork
prawns

Sample Recipes for the Whole Family

These sample recipes are designed to give you an idea how fresh, wholesome foods can be combined quickly and relatively simply to create healthy, filling, nutritious meals which are suitable for the whole family, but at the same time combine low-glycaemic index ingredients and super-foods. You'll see how delicious health can be!

These are not designed to be 'weight-loss' recipes. And that's because – as you'll have learned by now! – it's not about weight 'loss', but about nurturing yourself with love and balance, with a healthy mind in a healthy body, putting food into its proper context and eating the right amount at the correct time. That's the secret to a healthy weight and slim physique!

These recipes will certainly provide all the nurturing you need: body and mind, and taste buds too! Most importantly, they will give you optimum health and energy.

Just remember, always, not to overdo the portions and to enjoy your food with mindful moderation, taking your time… *'Taste it like you mean it!'* – that's what my children like to say!

Enjoy your meal!

Don't Forget the Condiments!

Nutty Pesto

(*Courtesy of designerhealthcenters.com, adapted.*)
What you need:
- fresh basil leaves
- 3 oz/80g chopped walnuts
- 4 cloves of peeled garlic
- 1½ oz/40g grated Parmesan cheese
- extra virgin olive oil to mix (until you are happy with the consistency)
- salt and pepper to taste

Blend the basil leaves, nuts, garlic and cheese together in a food processor. Add the oil slowly, mixing as you go. Stir in the salt and pepper.

If you don't have a food processor, finely chop the basil, use a mortar and pestle to grind the nuts, cheese and garlic together, and then transfer to a bowl and gradually stir in the oil. Finally season with salt and pepper to taste.

Lemon Vinaigrette

(*Courtesy of Erica Jones, adapted.*)
What you need:
- 2 fl. oz/60ml/¼ cup of fresh lemon juice
- a handful of lightly packed fresh Italian parsley leaves
- 2 cloves of garlic
- 2 teaspoons of finely grated lemon zest
- ½ teaspoon of salt
- ½ teaspoon of freshly ground black pepper
- 3 fl. oz/80 ml/1/3 cup extra virgin olive oil

Blend the lemon juice, parsley, garlic, lemon zest, salt and pepper in a blender. Gradually blend in the oil. Season the vinaigrette, to taste, with more salt and pepper.

If you don't have a blender, finely chop the parsley then shake the ingredients together in a large jam jar to blend.

Parsley-Mint Sauce

(*Courtesy of FoodNetwork.com, adapted.*)
What you need:
- a couple of handfuls of tightly packed fresh mint leaves
- a handful of tightly packed fresh flat-leaf parsley
- 6 cloves of garlic, chopped
- a small drizzle of honey or agave syrup
- 2 tablespoons of Dijon mustard
- 8 fl. oz/240ml/1 cup of olive oil
- water
- salt and freshly ground black pepper

Place the mint, parsley, and garlic in a food processor and process until coarsely chopped. Add the honey and mustard and process until combined. With the motor running, slowly add the olive oil until emulsified. Transfer the mixture to a bowl and whisk in a few tablespoons of cold water to thin to a sauce-like consistency. Season to taste with salt and pepper.

If you don't have a blender, finely chop the herbs, use a mortar and pestle to grind the garlic and mustard together and then transfer to a bowl and *very* gradually stir in the oil to achieve a sauce-like consistency. Finally season with salt and pepper to taste.

Cucumber Mint Yogurt Dip

(*Courtesy of wholeliving.com, adapted.*)
Serves 6 people.
What you need:
- 2 pots of 5 oz/150g each low-fat Greek-style yogurt
- a handful of mint leaves, coarsely chopped
- ½ cucumber, halved, peeled and finely chopped
- 1 teaspoon of white wine vinegar
- coarse salt and ground pepper
- cut vegetables, for serving (try cucumbers, peppers, or celery sticks)

In a medium bowl, combine the yogurt, mint, cucumber and vinegar, then season with the salt and pepper.

Can be kept in an airtight container in the fridge for up to three days.

Quick and Easy Tomato Sauce

(Courtesy of GuiltyKitchen.com, adapted.)

What you need:

- 1 clove of garlic, finely chopped
- 1 tablespoon of oil
- 1 tin of chopped tomatoes
- fresh or dried herbs: oregano, basil and marjoram, to taste

Heat the oil in small saucepan, add the garlic and stir for 1 minute. Add the tomato sauce and herbs. Simmer for 10–15 minutes. Serve with pasta, quinoa, or Portobello mushrooms (read more about quinoa - and how to cook it - at the end of this Recipe section, under *'Why Cut the (Low-GI!) Carbs?'*. There is a recipe for Portobello mushrooms under *'Viva Veggies'*).

Yummy, Useful, Low-GI, Filling Snacks (or Meal Replacements)

'Fast' Thin-Crust Veggie Pizza

(*Courtesy of designerhealthcenters.com, adapted.*)
Each pizza serves 1.
What you need:

- a brown tortilla-style wrap (brown rice recommended)
- pesto (try *Nutty Pesto,* under *'Don't Forget the Condiments'* at the beginning of this Recipe section.)
- either no-added sugar and low-salt pasta sauce* (you can make this at home)
- or *'Quick and Easy Tomato Sauce'* (just above).
- diced mushrooms
- diced red, orange or yellow peppers
- diced red onions
- any other vegetable you love (grated carrot is good)
- your choice of grated or crumbled cheese – goat's cheese is great!

This is a favourite snack at Designer Health Centers! You can enjoy this 'pizza' baked in the oven or served 'raw' and fresh.

Spread a layer of pesto on the wrap, followed by another layer of pasta sauce. Add the veggies to the wrap (to your personal taste). Top with grated cheese, or mix crumbled cheese like goat or feta in with the veggies, and pop the wrap in the oven for 10 to 15 minutes at 300°F, 150°C, gas mark 2 if you want it hot. Now you've got a delicious and healthy snack!

*Be careful with sugar in sauces. No sugar or at the very least low sugar (less than 2g) is what you should be aiming for.

Crunchy No-Bake Power Bars

(*Courtesy of Erica Jones, adapted.*)
Makes about 6, but can very easily be doubled or tripled, supplying the whole family with high-protein, 'good'-fat, high-fibre snacks.
What you need:
- two tablespoons of sunflower seeds
- 1½ oz/40g raw walnuts
- 1½ oz/40g raw pumpkin seeds
- 3 oz/80g raw almonds
- 3 oz/80g raw pecan nuts
- 1½ oz/40g unsweetened shredded coconut
- 1½ oz/40g almond nut butter
- a small knob of pure organic butter
- 1 teaspoon of vanilla extract
- 2 tablespoons of the sweetener xylitol* (in powder form)
- a pinch of salt (Himalayan salt, ideally)

Pulse the nuts, coconut and seeds in a food processor until the nuts are chopped, or roughly chop the lot if you haven't got a blender.

Over the very lowest heat (the goal is to keep as many nutrients intact, using as little heat as possible), gently melt the pure butter and nut butter. Stir until smooth.

Add vanilla extract, xylitol and sea salt, stirring until incorporated. Fold into nut mixture with a spatula.

Press into a baking tray lined with greaseproof paper using the back of a large spoon.

Quick set in the freezer for 20 minutes and later cut into bars (ready for quick snacks on the go). Store in the fridge.

*I recommend the brand Xylosweet. It can be found in many health food shops or online. Avoid xylitol that is made in China: there can be extra (but undesirable) additives in certain Chinese brands.

The DHC Granola Crunch

(*Courtesy of designerhealthcenters.com, adapted.*)
What you need:

- a pinch of cinnamon
- 2 tablespoons of coconut oil (from health food shops)
- ¾ tablespoon of xylitol powder (from health food shops)
- ½ teaspoon of vanilla essence
- 2 teaspoons of sesame seed
- 1¾ oz/50g of lightly toasted oats (for crunch) or whole uncooked oats (softer version)
- 11 oz/300g of assorted nuts (try walnuts, almonds and Brazil nuts)

It's ideal to soak the nuts first. Chop them up in a food processor or simply roughly chop them.

Then just mix all of the ingredients in a mixing bowl.

Mix together plain yogurt and this super granola for a quick snack, or for breakfast add almond or coconut milk!

Pumpkin Bars

(*Courtesy of elanaspantry.com, adapted.*)

- 4 oz/100g tinned pumpkin puree
- 3 tablespoons of agave syrup (lower GI than honey, available in most supermarkets now) or adapt to taste
- 2 eggs
- 4½ oz/120g almond flour (finely ground almonds)
- a pinch of sea salt
- ½ teaspoon of baking soda
- ¼ teaspoon of cinnamon
- ¼ teaspoon of nutmeg

Beat the eggs, then stir in the agave syrup and gradually combine the pumpkin *purée*. Fold in the dry ingredients until you have a well-combined batter.

Pour the batter into a greased baking dish and bake at 350°F, 180°C, gas mark 4 for 30–35 minutes until firm.

Satisfying that Sweet Tooth!

Yogurt *Parfait*

(*Courtesy of Self.com, adapted.*)
What you need:
- plain Greek yogurt, preferably low-fat
- chopped walnuts
- berries to taste

In a bowl, layer the yogurt, chopped walnuts and berries.

Papaya Yogurt *Parfait*

(*Courtesy of wholeliving.com, adapted.*)
Serves 6.
What you need:
- 3 small pots or one large (15 oz/400g) pot of plain low-fat Greek yogurt
- 6 teaspoons of agave syrup (lower GI) or a drizzle of honey
- 1½ teaspoons of grated lemon zest (unwaxed lemons are preferable), plus 1 tablespoon of lemon juice
- 1 knob of fresh ginger (about 2 inches/5 cm)
- 1 papaya, peeled, halved lengthwise, seeds discarded, cut into ¼ inch/1 cm cubes
- 1 punnet (7 oz/200g) fresh blackberries
- 1 punnet (7 oz/200g) fresh raspberries
- chopped fresh mint, plus sprigs for garnish
- 1¾ oz/50g granola

In a small bowl combine the yogurt, 3 teaspoons of syrup or honey and the lemon zest. Set aside.

Using the large holes of a box grater, grate the ginger (no need to peel) into a small bowl. Then squeeze it through a fine-meshed sieve or strainer placed over a medium bowl to get a total of 1 tablespoon of ginger juice. Discard the pulp. To the bowl with the juice, add the remaining 3 teaspoons of honey and the lemon juice; whisk to combine.

Add the papaya, blackberries and raspberries and toss gently to coat.

To serve: Spoon half the fruit and juice into six tall dessert glasses. Sprinkle the chopped mint over the fruit. Top with half the yogurt mixture and half the granola, and layer with the remaining fruit, yogurt and granola. Garnish with mint sprigs.

Healthy South Indian *Paysam* (Country Rice Pudding)

(*Courtesy of Laxmi Reddy.*)
What you need:
- 2½ pints/1½ litres of low-fat coconut milk or organic milk
- 4 oz/100g rice or wheat vermicelli (from Asian shops), alternatively coarse semolina, maize flour (cornmeal) or even Bulgar wheat
- 2½ oz/70g green raisins (from Asian shops) or sultanas as a substitute
- 1 teaspoon of ground ginger
- ½ teaspoon of ground cinnamon
- 2½ oz/70g flaked organic toasted almonds
- 2½ oz/70g cashew nuts, whole
- a pinch of ground cardamom or couple of cardamom cloves
- powdered xylitol* or agave syrup to sweeten, or a drizzle of raw organic honey
- rosewater if you can find it (specialist shops)

Toast the vermicelli (or substitute) lightly over a low heat in a wide heavy-based pan with a touch of ghee or unsalted organic pure butter until it smells nutty. Don't let it burn and try not to break the vermicelli strands. If toasting semolina or maize flour (cornmeal), stir constantly to prevent burning.

Remove from the heat and set aside on a plate. Toast the cashews and raisins lightly in a touch of ghee. Set aside.

Gently boil the milk in a large saucepan over the lowest heat with cardamom pods and spices added. Add the sweetener, nuts and raisins and finally the vermicelli or meal, stirring constantly so that no lumps can form, until the mixture thickens a little and the vermicelli or meal is cooked. Make sure that the mixture doesn't stick to the bottom of the pan and burn! Remember it will thicken even more as it cools.

Transfer to a serving dish and leave to cool. When cool, sprinkle with rosewater.

This is a filling, nutritious dish, usually eaten on special occasions with plain yogurt or fresh mango on the side.

*I recommend the brand Xylosweet. It can be found in many health food shops or online. Avoid xylitol that is made in China: there can be extra (but undesirable) additives in certain Chinese brands.

Brownies

(*Courtesy of* Now Eat This! *by Rocco Dispirito, adapted.*)
Makes about 12.

- unsalted organic butter for greasing the pan, plus an extra small knob
- 7 oz/200g black beans, rinsed and drained
- 1¾ oz/50g sweetened cocoa powder
- 1 tablespoon of espresso powder
- 1 organic egg
- 2 tablespoons of melted high-cocoa chocolate (70% and higher; Green & Black's is good)
- 2 tablespoons of sour cream
- 100g xylitol as a sugar substitute, or to taste*
- 1 teaspoon of vanilla extract

Preheat the oven to 350°F, 180°C, gas mark 4. Lightly wipe an 8x8 inch/20x20 cm glass baking dish with butter or cooking oil spray.

Combine the beans, cocoa powder, espresso powder and egg in the bowl of a food processor. Process until the mixture is smooth, about 2 minutes, scraping down the bowl halfway through. If you don't have a food processor, a hand-held mixer and sturdy bowl are fine!

Melt the chocolate very slowly over a *bain-marie* (in a shatter-proof bowl over simmering boiling water), then gently stir in the sour cream, the butter, the powdered xylitol and the vanilla essence. Mix until all of the ingredients are combined and you get a batter.

Pour the batter into the baking dish and smooth the top with a spatula.

Bake for 28 to 30 minutes, turning the dish halfway through the baking time. When it is cooked, a toothpick inserted in the centre should come out with soft batter clinging to it.

Let the brownies cool completely in the baking dish on a wire rack. Then cut into 12 squares and serve. Refrigerate leftovers – if there are any!

*I recommend the brand Xylosweet. It can be found in many health food shops or online. Avoid xylitol that is made in China: there can be extra (but undesirable) additives in certain Chinese brands.

Classic Carrot Cake with Creamy Coconut Frosting

(*Courtesy of* The Gluten-Free Almond Flour Cookbook, *by Elana Amsterdam,* *adapted*.)

- 12 oz/350g blanched almond flour (or finely ground almonds)
- 2 teaspoons of sea salt
- 1 teaspoons of baking soda
- 1 tablespoon of ground cinnamon
- 1 teaspoon of ground nutmeg
- 4 fl. oz/120 ml almond oil
- 4 tablespoons of low-GI agave syrup
- 5 large organic eggs
- 15½ oz/450g grated carrots
- 5 oz/150g raisins
- 5 oz/150g walnuts, coarsely chopped

Preheat the oven to 325°F, 160°C, gas mark 3. Grease two 9 inch/22 cm cake tins with a spray of oil or a light rub of organic unsalted butter and dust with almond flour.

In a large bowl, combine the almond flour, salt, baking soda, cinnamon and nutmeg.

In a medium bowl, whisk together the oil, syrup and eggs.

Fold the wet ingredients into the almond flour mixture until thoroughly combined. Fold in the carrots, raisins and walnuts. Scoop the batter into the prepared cake tins.

Bake for 30 to 35 minutes until a toothpick inserted into the centre of the cake comes out clean. Let the cakes cool in the pans for one hour.

For the Coconut Frosting:
- 8 fl. oz/240 ml unsweetened coconut milk
- agave syrup to taste
- a pinch of sea salt
- 2 tablespoons of arrowroot powder or thickening starch
- 1 tablespoon of water

In a medium saucepan, bring the coconut milk, syrup and salt to the boil, stirring to combine.

Whisk the ingredients together, then decrease the heat and simmer for 8–10 minutes, stirring frequently.

In a small bowl, dissolve the arrowroot powder or thickener in water, stirring to make a paste.

Raise the heat under the saucepan to medium high. Add the arrowroot paste to the coconut mixture, whisking constantly until the mixture thickens (about 1 minute). Remove the pan from the heat and stir until smooth.

Place in the freezer for 30 to 35 minutes until the frosting solidifies and turns an opaque white. Remove from the freezer and whip with a handheld mixer until thick and fluffy. Use to frost the carrot cake. It can also serve as filling between the two cake layers.

The frosting can be stored in a glass jar for up to 3 days.

Nice Bit o' Fish!

Pacific Cod with Roasted Shiitake Mushrooms

(*Courtesy of wholeliving.com, adapted.*)
Serves 4.
What you need:

- 2 packets of fresh shiitake mushrooms, stems removed, halved if large
- 4 tablespoons of sesame seed oil
- 4 sprigs of fresh rosemary
- coarse sea salt
- ground black pepper
- 4 large Pacific cod or halibut fillets
- 1 tablespoon of fresh lemon juice
- 1 tablespoon of Dijon mustard
- 2 tablespoons of finely chopped parsley

Preheat oven to 450°F, 230°C, gas mark 8.

On a large baking tray, toss the mushrooms with 2 tablespoons of oil and rosemary; season with salt and pepper. Roast until tender and browned, tossing occasionally.

Push the mushrooms to the sides of the pan, place the cod in the centre and season with salt and pepper. Roast until opaque throughout (8–10 minutes). To check if the fish is cooked, insert a fork then test the temperature of the fork on your wrist. If it's cool, the fish is still rare; if it's warm, the fish is almost cooked.

Meanwhile, in a small bowl, whisk together remaining the remaining oil, lemon juice, mustard and parsley; season with salt and pepper. Serve with or over the cod.

White Fish with Lemon Vinaigrette and Butter Beans

(Courtesy of designer healthcenters.com, adapted.)
Serves 6 – perfect for a family meal.
It's best to make the lemon vinaigrette first (under *'Don't Forget the Condiments!'* at the start of the recipe section).
What you need:
- oil: sesame seed oil is nice, or light olive, or oil with garlic and ginger
- ½ cup of red onions, diced (¼ cup if you don't love onions)
- 1 large head of radicchio lettuce, coarsely chopped, or a small red cabbage
- 1 can butter beans, drained and rinsed
- 4 fl. oz/100 ml fish broth, or *consommé* or vegetable broth if preferred
- salt and freshly ground black pepper
- 6 large white fish fillets (cod or tilapia or coley or similar)
- flour, almond flour or ground oats, for dusting

Heat 2 tablespoons of oil in a heavy-bottomed pan, over a medium heat. Add the onions and *sauté* until tender and transparent. Add the red cabbage or radicchio and *sauté* until wilted. Add the beans and broth and cook until the beans are heated through, stirring often. Season the red cabbage mixture to taste, with salt and freshly ground black pepper.

Meanwhile, heat 3 tablespoons of oil in a non-stick frying pan over a medium-high heat. Sprinkle the fillets with salt and pepper and dust the fillets in flour to coat completely. Shake off the excess flour and fry until they are golden brown and just cooked through (about 3 minutes per side).

Spoon the radicchio mixture over the centre of the plates. Top with the fillets. Drizzle the vinaigrette over and serve immediately.

Salmon Salad

(*Courtesy of foodnetwork.com, adapted.*)

Serves 4.

What you need:

- 4 pieces of cooked salmon, chilled
- 3 stalks of finely diced celery
- 1 finely diced red onion
- 2 tablespoons of fresh dill, minced
- 2 tablespoons of capers, drained
- 2 tablespoons of raspberry vinegar
- 2 tablespoons of olive oil
- ½ teaspoon of sea salt, ground
- ½ teaspoon of freshly ground black pepper
- chopped romaine lettuce, or mixed greens

Flake the salmon, removing any skin and bones, and place in a bowl. Add the celery, red onion, dill, capers, raspberry vinegar, olive oil, salt and pepper. Season to taste. Mix well and serve cold or at room temperature over about lettuce or mixed greens.

Good Old British Fish Fingers – Natasha Reddy's Healthy Designer Version!

What you need:
- 5 oz/150g ground almonds (not too fine) – semolina or rice flour are also good if you are allergic to nuts
- 1 organic free-range egg, beaten
- fresh chopped coriander or flat-leaf parsley
- 1lb/500g fresh white firm fish like cod, alternatively fresh tuna, cut into ½ inch-thick fingers
- light olive oil or sunflower seed oil

Mix together the ground almonds and herbs on a flat plate and season with a little sea salt and fresh black pepper. Gently rub the fish with the beaten egg using a spoon, so that it's damp but not too sticky. Roll the fish in the almond mixture, enough to coat it.

Heat the oil in a good heavy non-stick pan over a low flame, but not until it smokes. Carefully place the fish fingers in the pan with a spatula, turning until they are golden and toasty, being careful not to burn them. To check if the fish is cooked, insert a fork then test the temperature of the fork on your wrist. If it's cool, the fish is still rare; if it's warm, the fish is almost cooked.

The fingers should take 5 minutes or so to cook per side, but this depends on the fish used. You can also brown them in the pan then transfer them to a baking tray in the oven to finish off, at 450°F, 230°C, gas mark 8 for 5 minutes or so.

Almond Encrusted Salmon or Trout

(*Courtesy* Bon Appétit, *Epicurious.com, adapted.*)
Serves 6.
What you need:

- ½ oz/20g organic butter
- 2 medium leeks, prepared and halved, very thinly sliced (only use the tender white and light green parts)
- 3 tablespoons of fresh lemon juice
- 1 pot *crème fraiche*
- 5 oz/150g sliced almonds, further chopped
- a handful of chopped fresh parsley
- 1 tablespoon grated lemon peel
- ½ teaspoon of salt
- a pinch of ground black pepper
- 2 oz/60g almond flour or finely ground almonds
- 6 skinless and boneless salmon or 'salmon' (pink) trout fillets (avoid farmed if possible)
- 1 large egg, beaten
- 2 teaspoons of sesame or light oil

Melt the butter in a large heavy-based saucepan over a medium-high heat. Add the leeks; *sauté* for 2 minutes. Reduce the heat to low; cover and cook until the leeks are very tender, stirring occasionally (about 20 minutes). Increase the heat to medium; add the lemon juice and stir until the liquid evaporates (about 1 minute). Mix in the cream. Simmer until slightly reduced (about 2 minutes). Cool slightly. Season to taste, with salt and freshly ground black pepper.

Mix the almonds, parsley, lemon peel, ½ teaspoon salt and pinch of pepper on a flat plate. Place the flour on another plate. Sprinkle the salmon with salt and pepper. Dust the fish in the flour, shaking off any excess. Then lightly brush one flank of the fish fillet with the beaten egg and press this brushed flank into the almond mixture, pressing lightly to adhere. Place the fish, nutty coating up, on a baking tray.

Melt a knob of butter with 1 tablespoon of oil in a large heavy-bottomed pan over a medium heat. Place the fish in the pan, almond-coated side down, and cook until the crust is brown (about 5 minutes). Turn the fish over until cooked through and opaque in the centre (about 5 minutes). To check if the fish is cooked, insert a fork then test the temperature of the fork on your wrist. If it's cool, the fish is still rare; if it's warm, the fish is almost cooked.

Transfer your lovely fish to plates. Reheat the sauce, stirring over medium heat. Spoon around the salmon and serve!

Baked Tilapia

(*Courtesy of Erica Jones, adapted.*)
What you need:
- 2 large tilapia, filleted
- juice of 1 lemon
- 1 teaspoon of sea salt
- chopped fresh parsley
- 1 teaspoon of finely chopped garlic
- olive oil

Lightly coat the bottom of a glass casserole or baking dish with oil to prevent sticking. Lay the tilapia filets in the dish and sprinkle with the lemon juice. Add the sea salt, garlic and parsley flakes.

Bake in the oven at 400°F, 200°C, gas mark 5–6 for 15–20 mins or until the fish is cooked through. To check if the fish is cooked, insert a fork then test the temperature of the fork on your wrist. If it's cool, the fish is still rare; if it's warm, the fish is almost cooked.

Give Me my Meat!

Ginger Chicken Stir-Fry

(*Courtesy of Erica Jones, adapted.*)
Serves 2.
What you need:
- quinoa or brown rice (read more about quinoa - and how to cook it - at the end of this Recipe section, under *'Why Cut the (Low-GI!) Carbs?'*)
- 2 cups of water
- 5 oz/150g red peppers
- 2 large red onions
- 1 tablespoon of grated ginger
- 5 oz/150g mushrooms
- 2 chicken breasts chopped into bite-sized strips
- light olive oil
- salt and pepper to taste
- a squeeze of lime juice

Pre-season the chicken strips with the ground sea salt and freshly ground black pepper. Cook them in a frying pan with a dash of oil, along with the onions, red peppers, mushrooms and ginger.

Once the chicken is cooked throughout, serve the stir-fry on a bed of quinoa or brown rice with a squeeze of lime juice.

Pepper Steak

(*Courtesy of* Now Eat This! *by Rocco Dispirito, adapted.*)
Serves 4.
What you need:

- 2 or 3 large red and green ('bell') peppers for frying, cut into quarters lengthwise
- 4 slices of organic beef tenderloin
- sea salt and freshly ground black pepper
- olive oil
- 1 red onion, thinly sliced
- 5 garlic cloves, finely chopped
- 3 tablespoons of balsamic vinegar
- 12 fl. oz/350 ml chicken broth or bouillon
- 3 tablespoons of arrowroot, or starch thickener like potato starch
- 4 fl. oz/120 ml Quick and Easy Tomato Sauce (*see p.000*)
- 4 fl. oz/120 ml almond or coconut milk
- a handful of chopped fresh chives

Place the peppers into a small saucepan with a spoonful of water and a spoonful of oil. Put the lid on and turn the heat to high. This will 'char' the peppers, so keep on shaking them to cook them evenly until the skins are slightly blackened.

Heat a large heavy-bottomed pan over a medium-high heat. Season the steaks with salt and pepper. When the skillet is hot, add one tablespoon of oil. Add the steaks and *sauté* until golden brown (about 4 minutes each side). Transfer them to a platter and cover to keep warm.

Add the sliced onion to the pan you cooked the steaks in. *Sauté* until the onions become tender (about 5 minutes). Add the garlic and *sauté* for 1 minute. Add the vinegar, mixing in with a wooden spoon.

In a small bowl, whisk the chicken broth and arrowroot or potato starch, then stir it into the pan and simmer. Stir in the tomato sauce and coconut or almond milk. Add the peppers and continue simmering for 1 minute. Stir in the chives.

Season with salt and pepper to taste, spoon the sauce over the steaks and serve!

Spicy Chicken Breasts with Parsley-Mint Sauce

(*Courtesy of Erica Jones, adapted.*)

Serves 4.

What you need:

- 1 tablespoon of light 'garam masala' or curry powder, if desired
- 1 tablespoon of smoked paprika
- 2 teaspoons of cumin seeds, ground
- 2 teaspoons of mustard seeds, ground
- 2 teaspoons of fennel seeds, ground
- 1 teaspoon of coarsely ground black pepper
- 2 teaspoons of salt
- 4 large (boneless) chicken breasts
- light olive oil
- parsley-mint sauce (*see p.000; it's best to make this first*)

Preheat your grill to medium high (or use a heavy-based pan on the hob at medium heat).

Mix together the paprika, cumin, mustard, fennel, pepper and salt in a small bowl to create a 'rub' for the meat. Brush the chicken with a few teaspoons of oil on both sides. Rub the breasts with some of the rub and place on the grill (or pan), rub side down.

Cook until golden brown (about 4–5 minutes). Turn the breasts over and continue cooking until just cooked through (4–5 minutes).

Transfer the chicken to a platter and immediately drizzle with some of the parsley-mint sauce. Serve with pleasure!

Herby Lamb Chops

Serves 2.

What you need:

- olive oil
- 4 lamb chops
- ground sea salt and freshly ground black pepper
- a splash of full-bodied red wine
- 1 clove garlic, minced
- 1 tablespoon of fresh thyme leaves, minced
- 1 teaspoon of fresh rosemary leaves, chopped
- 1 teaspoon of fresh parsley leaves, chopped
- 1 tablespoon fresh chives, minced

Preheat a heavy-bottomed pan or grill pan over medium-high heat and add a splash of oil. Season each side of the lamb chops well with salt and pepper to taste. Sear one side of the lamb. Lower the heat to medium and then turn the lamb over and sear that side too.

Add the garlic and fresh herbs until they are aromatic and cooked. Finally add the splash of red wine and reduce it completely. Pair with veggies and boiled new potatoes for a tasty dinner!

Get to Work on an Egg!

Pepper and Basil Frittata

(*Courtesy of* Now Eat This! *by Rocco Dispirito, adapted.*)
Serves 6.

- What you need:
- 2 teaspoons of light olive oil
- 11 oz/300g cauliflower florets
- • ½ medium-sized courgette (zucchini), cut in half lengthwise and sliced into half moons
- 2 garlic cloves, finely chopped
- ground sea salt and freshly ground black pepper
- 5 oz/150g jar of roasted red pepper strips (not oil packed) – or pre-cook them yourself
- 4 oz/100g grated Parmigiano (Reggiano) cheese
- a handful of chopped fresh basil
- 6 eggs
- romaine lettuce (roughly chopped) or mixed greens

Preheat the oven to 475°F, 240°C, gas mark 9. Heat a heavy-bottomed pan over a medium-high heat. Once the pan is hot, add one spoonful of oil, then the cauliflower and courgettes. *Sauté* the vegetables for 5 minutes, then add the garlic and salt and pepper to taste. Cover the pan and reduce the heat to low. Continue to cook until the vegetables are tender (another 5 minutes). Add the red pepper strips to the pan and stir to combine. Raise the heat to medium-high.

Whisk the cheese, basil and eggs together in a medium-sized bowl. Season the mixture with salt and pepper to taste. Stir the egg mixture into the *sauté* pan. Continue to stir as the eggs begin to solidify. When there are large curds but the mixture is still wet, flatten it slightly with a spatula and stop stirring. Cook undisturbed for 1 minute, then transfer the pan to the hot oven.

Bake the frittata for about 8 minutes or until the eggs are completely set. Remove the pan from the oven and give it a good shake to loosen the frittata. Invert a plate on top of the frittata and flip it over!

In a medium-sized bowl, mix the romaine lettuce with 1 teaspoon of olive oil and 2 tablespoons of cheese. Season the salad with salt and pepper to taste. Cut the frittata into wedges and serve hot or at room temperature with the romaine salad as a side dish.

Florentine Omelette

(Courtesy of kitchendaily.com, adapted.)
Serves 2.
What you need:
- 2 eggs
- 2 egg whites
- 3 tablespoons of water
- 1 teaspoon of dried mixed Italian herbs
- ¼ teaspoon of salt
- 2 tablespoons of light olive oil
- 9 oz/250g mushrooms, sliced
- 1 large onion, chopped
- 1 red ('bell') pepper, chopped
- 1 clove of garlic, finely chopped
- 11 oz/300g spinach leaves, washed and roughly chopped
- 2 oz/60g shredded lower-fat hard mozzarella cheese (or Edam)

In a medium-sized bowl, whisk the eggs, egg whites, water, Italian herbs and salt. Add some of the oil to a heavy-bottomed pan and place over a medium-high heat. Add the mushrooms, onion, pepper and garlic and cook, stirring often, for about 4 minutes. Add the spinach and cook for a further minute, or until the spinach is wilted. Place aside in a bowl and cover.

Adjust the heat to medium and add another spoonful of oil. Pour in half of the egg mixture and cook for 2 minutes or until the bottom begins to set, lifting the edges with a spatula so the uncooked mixture floods into the bottom of pan and cooks too. Cook until set but still soft and fluffy (be careful not to overcook: it must not be hard and rubbery!) Sprinkle with half of the vegetable mixture and half of the cheese. Cook gently on the lowest flame until the cheese melts, then fold in half with the spatula and serve immediately with crusty wholegrain bread.

Repeat previous steps to prepare a second omelette – it is easier to cook two medium-sized ones than one huge one.

Crust-less and Quick Quiche

(Courtesy of allrecipes.com, adapted.)
Serves 6.
What you need:
- 8 rashers of lean bacon
- 4 organic free-range eggs
- chopped onions
- chopped red peppers
- 4 oz/100g shredded cheese of your choice
- 12 fl. oz/350 ml of sugar-free almond or coconut milk
- a knob of organic unsalted butter
- 4 oz/100g brown rice or almond flour
- sea salt and freshly ground black pepper to taste

Preheat your oven to 350°F, 180°C, gas mark 4.

Cook the bacon, then crumble it and set aside. Lightly grease a 9 inch/22 cm pie mould with the butter. Layer the bottom of the mould with the cheese and the crumbled bacon.

Mix together the eggs, onions, peppers, milk, flour, salt and pepper and lightly whisk together until blended, then pour over the bacon and cheese. If you're a real cheese lover, add some shredded cheese to the top of the dish before it goes in the oven.

Bake for about 35 minutes until cooked throughout.

Viva Veggies!

Dr Jones' Zucchini (Courgette) Pasta

(Courtesy of Dr Isaac Jones.)

Calculate the quantity of zucchini (courgette) based on one medium to large vegetable per person.

If you have a food processor, you can hook up the julienne or mandolin attachment for perfectly formed noodles. If you're like most people, you probably don't have one, but you can easily use a vegetable peeler or a knife instead! The peeler method will give you long flat noodles, and if using a knife, just cut the zucchini into long, thin slices.

The 'noodles' won't need to cook long. Just cover them with a spaghetti sauce of your choice and cook over medium heat until heated throughout. Don't overcook the zucchini, though – it will lose its texture and become more like steamed veg!

Stuffed Portobello Mushrooms on Quinoa

(*Courtesy of GuiltyKitchen.com, adapted.*)
Serves 2.
What you need:
- 2 large Portobello (big, flat!) mushrooms
- ½ small onion, diced
- 1 clove garlic, minced
- a glug of light olive oil
- 3 oz/75g sun-dried tomatoes, chopped
- 2 mushrooms, diced
- 9 oz/250g baby spinach leaves, roughly chopped or torn
- 3 oz/75g goat's cheese or feta
- 1 oz/30g grated Parmesan cheese
- romaine lettuce or mixed greens

Preheat the oven to 375°F, 190°C, gas mark 5. *Sauté* the onions and garlic with the oil in a heavy-bottomed pan over a medium heat until the onions begin to turn translucent. Remove the stems from the mushrooms and chop. Add the tomatoes and diced mushroom stems to the onions in the pan and *sauté* for 5 minutes.

Add the spinach leaves to the pan. *Sauté* until completely cooked, remove from heat and stir in the Parmesan cheese. Set aside.

Place the Portobello mushroom 'caps' on a baking tray and pile the spinach mix onto them equally. Top with crumbled goat or feta cheese and bake for 20–25 minutes.

Serve on a bed of quinoa (*see p.000*) and tomato sauce.

Harvest Salad

(Courtesy of Cindy Jindrich, adapted.)

What you need:

- 11 oz/300g chopped tomatoes
- 5 oz/150g thinly sliced radishes
- 7 oz/200g cubed cucumber
- ½ to 2 very thinly sliced red onion(s), depending on the strength and size of the onion and your taste
- 1 large avocado, cut into large chunks
- red wine vinegar, to taste
- fresh dill
- sea salt, ground
- freshly ground black pepper
- a glug of good olive oil

Mix all the non-veg. ingredients together until well blended to make a dressing and gently toss with the salad vegetables. Enjoy with crusty wholegrain bread.

Keralan Aromatic Green Beans

(Courtesy of Laxmi Reddy.)
What you need:
- 1lb/500g fine green beans, trimmed and cut or left whole
- walnut oil, chilli or garlic or plain light olive oil
- desiccated coconut or fresh grated coconut
- mustard seeds
- fresh red chillies if wanted.

Pre-steam the green beans until *al dente*. Heat the oil but not so it smokes. Cook the mustard seeds until they 'pop' to release their flavour, being careful to cover the pan. Add the chillies whole but don't burn them!
Add the beans to the pan and cook until a little browned, then add the coconut and stir rapidly until it smells aromatic.
Serve with a wedge of lemon to squeeze over.
Super with fish curry, or steamed fish of any type.

Grecian Spinach *Sauté*

(Courtesy of Erica Jones, adapted.)
Serves 2.
What you need:
- 1 tablespoon of light olive oil
- ½ small red onion, sliced into thin rings
- 1lb/500g of fresh baby spinach, washed thoroughly
- ½ teaspoon of grated lemon peel (unwaxed lemons are preferable)
- salt and freshly ground black pepper
- 1 oz/30g crumbled feta cheese
- 1½ oz/40g diced black olives

Heat a large pan with a lid over medium heat. Add oil, diced black olives and sliced red onion. *Sauté* until the onion starts to wilt. Add the spinach and quickly *sauté* again for 2 to 3 minutes. Add the lemon peel and season with the salt and pepper. Cook for a few seconds more to release the flavour, then pop in the crumbled feta and stir in. Transfer to serving dish and serve immediately.

Chunky Gazpacho Soup

(Courtesy of foodnetwork.com, adapted.)
Serves 4 to 6.
What you need:

- 1 cucumber, halved but not peeled
- 2 red peppers, cored and seeded
- 4 plum tomatoes
- 1 red onion
- 3 garlic cloves, finely chopped
- 3 cups of tomato juice
- a splash of white wine vinegar
- a dash of good olive oil
- sea salt, ground
- freshly ground black pepper

Roughly chop the cucumbers, peppers, tomatoes and red onions. Combine them in a large bowl and add the garlic, tomato juice, vinegar, olive oil, salt and pepper. Mix well and chill before serving. The longer gazpacho sits, the more the flavour develops!

Serve with some nice crusty wholegrain bread and a scrape of organic unsalted butter!

Why Cut the (Low-GI!) Carbs?

Tomato and Shallot Spaghetti

(*Courtesy of* The Alkaline Diet Recipe Book *by Ross Bridgeford, adapted.*)
What you need:
- 1 tablespoon of light olive oil
- 1 spring onion, finely chopped
- 1 garlic clove, finely chopped
- 4 ½ oz/125g sun-blushed tomatoes, roughly chopped
- a handful of cauliflower 'flowers'
- 1 large handful of baby spinach
- 1 large handful of rocket
- 1 handful each of chives, parsley and basil, all finely chopped
- ½ lemon, juice only
- 9 oz/250g spaghetti, cooked, preferably pulse-based or wholegrain. Cooked chick peas are also nice as an alternative, as is cous-cous or Bulgar wheat for a Middle Eastern twist.

Prepare the pasta according to the packet guidelines. While it is cooking away, prepare your vegetables. Chop the cauliflower so that it is quite fine, and if you haven't yet done so, finely chop the garlic, spring onion and herbs.
Heat the oil and very gently fry the spring onion, garlic and tomatoes. Don't let anything brown or burn in the slightest – you're almost just warming it up!
Throw the herbs and leaves into the pan just to get a slight coating of the oil and flavour and then squeeze over the lemon juice.
Either mix into the pasta or serve on top.

Canadian Baked Potato

(*Courtesy of Erica Jones.*)
Rinse a jacket potato, prick several times and bake at 350°F, 180°C, gas mark 4, for about one hour. (Please don't use aluminium foil because the metal can leach into the potato at such high temperatures.)
Once the potato is soft, add butter and cinnamon, or simply your favourite topping!

Quinoa

(Acknowledgements to designerhealthcenters.com.)
Meet quinoa (pronounced 'keen-owa'), the healthy pseudo-grain! Quinoa is an amino acid protein seed from South America. It is full of health benefits due to the fact that it is made up of all nine essential amino acids. It is also high in protein and lysine, so beneficial for tissue growth and restoration. In addition it is an excellent source of magnesium, riboflavin and manganese, all of which are excellent for fighting migraines, diabetes and heart disease. Quinoa is a true super-food!

Use quinoa as a substitute for brown rice in some of your favourite conventional dishes. My young children have come to love it! Nowadays you can buy it in all major British supermarkets, as it has become more of a mainstream ingredient.

How to Cook It

Rinse the quinoa three times with plain water, draining it as much as possible. Its natural coating, called saponin, can make it taste ever so slightly bitter and soaking helps to reduce this.

In a medium-sized saucepan, mix the quinoa, the recommended amount of water (follow the packet instructions) or vegetable stock or bouillon for a tastier flavour, half a teaspoon of salt if not using stock or bouillon, herbs to taste and a scrape of butter. Bring to the boil, cover and lower to simmer for 15–20 minutes. You can tell when it is cooked, as the tiny 'curls' start to separate from the grains. Do not overcook, as it will become unpleasantly mushy! The texture should be that of cous-cous.

Remove from heat and allow to rest for 5 minutes. Fluff with a fork before serving.

Quinoa can also be cooked very nicely in a rice-cooker, 1 cup of quinoa to 1½ cups of water.

Eat as an accompaniment to meat and fish dishes.

Afterword

So …what now? This is for life, so how do you keep it all going?

Any change which is going to have long-term effects must logically be a long-term commitment. Either you want to make the most of yourself and your life or you don't, and the only course of action which is really effective, reaps results and doesn't backtrack is one where you put in the effort each and every day over a sustained period of time. It need not be an impossible amount of exertion, either. It stands to reason that it's easier (and more productive) to apply yourself a little every day rather than go for a mammoth exertion all at once! Weaving a healthy, balanced attitude to diet and fitness into your everyday lifestyle and routine might take a little concentration and a touch of discipline at the outset. However, as time goes on, it will become more and more of a way of life.

As we know by now, anything which is too difficult (or not enjoyable enough) will never motivate most of us for very long, so we aren't talking sacrifices here or rigid regimes!

Do you remember we talked about the Power of Seven? Making health and fitness a way of life can also be summed up in seven points, one to ponder over (or to practise) every day of every week:

1. Eat only when you are hungry.
2. Stop when you are full.
3. Eat slowly.
4. Make sensible dietary choices for yourself and your family.
5. Take regular exercise which you enjoy.
6. Have a balanced and calm attitude.
7. Respect yourself both physically and emotionally.

None of these are difficult in themselves – hardly as difficult as cutting out chocolate from your diet forever. Personally, I could never do that unless I had an allergy to it!

Just remember the alterative: fighting hunger and deprivation and the restrictive, frustrating regime of a traditional 'slimming diet' and that feeling of 'I can't wait for this to end'!

Granted, following the advice in this book will naturally take a certain amount of energy, a little bit of awareness and concentration every day. After all, you don't get anywhere in life without a little bit of endeavour, but it's all a small price to pay if you see the process as a road you're driving down to reach a destination – and you're so excited about getting there!

And why not be excited when the end result is a slim, fit body and a healthy mind, freedom from worrying about body image and ongoing happiness with the way you are right into the future!

And while you're on the way, here's a couple of things to note...

Treat Yourself

Optimism is self-reinforcing and self-creating. Basically, happiness breeds happiness and optimism breeds optimism.

Those who have children or can remember what it is like to be a child will know the power of a treat. Unfortunately, as we know, once we are adult, things get rather blown out of proportion and we often abuse treats rather than use them to provide the pleasure and reward that they gave us in our childhood.

However, there is absolutely nothing *wrong* with using food as a treat. Many parents nowadays are frightened about doing so because they worry that their children might grow up to be compulsive eaters or unable to control their appetites. But there are always two sides to the coin. If we truly learn to love food for what it is and are able to appreciate its nurturing abilities, as well as enjoy its taste and texture, then we will learn how to respect it and have a balanced relationship with it.

I love a treat. Allowing yourself a treat from time to time means allowing yourself to accept the wondrous experience of delicious food – whether your thing is sweet, oily, fried or savoury – without an ounce of guilt. To learn to sit quietly alone, or with friends, and concentrate fully on the taste and texture and fragrance of something you truly enjoy, *without* guilt or recrimination, is to treat yourself, to tell yourself that *you are worth it*. It is proof that you value yourself, and that you trust that you are strong and balanced, able to appreciate a 'treat' wholeheartedly without feeling out of control and guilty.

This is why the strong, slim, confident and elegant women I know are totally partial to a croissant with their cappuccino from time to time. They know that the balanced relationship they have towards food and, most importantly, the respect they have for themselves will allow them to 'treat' themselves occasionally and still have the figure they desire!

And, after all, one croissant, or ice-cream, or dessert, or piece of chocolate never made anyone visibly fatter! But *guilt does make many people fatter.* It leads to addiction and lack of attention: if you are so consumed by the guilt you feel when you are eating a croissant, you will only taste the guilt and never the croissant! That way, no number of croissants (substitute your thing) will ever truly fulfil you. So beware.

Be the person who deserves a treat, not to cheer yourself up because you're *not* what you want to be, but because you *are* who you want to be!

Dressing into your Dreams

People talk about a 'fat' and a 'thin' wardrobe, but scrap this concept immediately! To become slim, you need to *feel* slim, *act* slim and, most importantly, *think* slim! If you're feeling so fat that you've had to put on your 'fat' clothes, you'll no doubt be suffering a lack of self-esteem and guilt – and first thing in the morning, too! Needless to say, this is unlikely to encourage you to think and behave like a slim person during the day.

You know now that your mind creates whatever you conceive and believe, so by thinking you're overweight, or fat, or unattractive, you will dress, stand and move accordingly. And, most crucially, you will *eat* accordingly ('I've already got a few pounds overweight, so I might as well finish off these chocolates to cheer myself up…') You are also likely to dress in baggy, forgiving clothes which don't give you the impetus to lose weight and which do hide a multitude of sins.

However, if you 'think slim', you will start to stand taller, dress in a more tailored fashion and behave like the poised, slim, elegant person you're planning to become! Have you ever noticed how when some people have even lost just a little weight, they start to 'feel' slimmer simply because of the success they're having? And how that feeling of success really changes the way they behave: suddenly they seem to have loads of positive energy! Well, these are the people who generally go on to greater weight-loss success! And the most important change is really what they've done to their own thoughts: they've changed the voice in their heads from 'I'm fat!' to 'I'm getting slimmer!'

So what I want you to do is start to 'dress slim' too. This sends an important message to the unconscious mind. Now of course I don't mean immediately going for skinny jeans if that's not what you'll fit into or look good in, but dressing in something that makes you *feel* slimmer. How about working around your best assets to make the most of them? Maybe you've got a particularly striking face? Maybe your tumbling mane is what people comment on? How about wearing a colour that offsets your eyes? What's your best feature: your arms, your neck, your bust? If you don't feel body confident at all, how about choosing a striking pattern or necklace that shows your love of colour or funky taste (colours can really help to cheer you up and give you a boost, even if only on a nice bright bangle or scarf, or tie for the men)? Knowing simply that you can be proud of a part of yourself, or of your outfit, will give you a confidence boost, and remember that *confidence begets confidence*! If you feel more confident and energetic than yesterday, you'll set yourself up to do the right things to feel even more confident and energetic tomorrow!

So, instead of dressing in clothes that dent your confidence and energy by reminding you that you're not the shape you want to be, try shaking things up and going to the next level by buying something which shouts that you feel *good*, which shouts that you're *en route* to becoming *slimmer*, which shouts newfound *confidence*! Be bold: throw away your ugliest, baggiest clothes. Start to *dress* confident and *dress* slimmer, and before you know it, you'll have lost those few pounds.

Do remember to wear something that you *do* fit into, though! There's no point in squeezing into a size that's too small and feeling so depressed about the tight fit that you fall onto the croissants for comfort. Low-slung skinny jeans are also not a good look if you've got a little belly and you're not 17 years old any longer – hanging out over low-cut jeans is not a sexy look!

Something well-cut and possibly tailored, however, can actually help you to look slimmer. Note also that something a little body-skimming (in a good way) can provide a visible and immediate incentive not to overeat. It's an old trick. Think of those actresses at the Oscars who probably can't get away with eating too much party food in their body-skimming frocks!

On the other hand, inmates in one correctional facility in the US were reported gaining 20–25 pounds during a jail sentence of an average of six months, despite having access to exercise facilities. They blamed the baggy orange jumpsuits they had to wear – these prison outfits were so loose-fitting there was no way to gauge weight gain. Without their usual 'signal clothes' – usually waistbands and belts, which we use to gauge our current weight – inmates had no idea they were gaining 'prison pounds'![1]

Tip: If you have a lot of weight to lose, buy a new pair of your favourite item of clothing *every time* you drop to a smaller size and give away the old size! Don't worry about the monetary cost – it'll more than pay for itself in confidence, believe me.

Do you know why what I call 'dressing into your dreams' actually works? Because when you're thinking – and dressing – the part, you'll start to act the part and behave accordingly! You'll eat healthily and not to excess, realizing that to overindulge doesn't fit either your new image or your new ambitions. *You'll start to eat with dignity if you feel more dignified!* You will also start to have a taste of what it feels like to feel confident – confident enough to go to the next level and wear something you're going to feel good in – and feel slimmer in!

Our unconscious mind is very good at justifying things, and it likes to be right. So, if you're wearing baggy clothes, well, that's enough justification for continuing to snack and overeat because you can 'hide' your guilt under your clothes, whether or not you'd consciously think of it that way. But if, on the other hand, you're wearing slimmer clothes, your unconscious mind will start to direct you to behave in a way that justifies you wearing them: you will start to take care that you don't overfill your stomach and ruin the line of those nice new jeans – and you'll no longer have the excuse that you can hide under baggy layers! No more hiding extra servings under voluminous clothes!

If you wear baggy clothes for cultural reasons – the two-piece shalwar kameez, for example, or an Indian sari – you can still gauge your size with undergarments or the fit of the blouse, and feel good about purchasing a smaller size. Even women who wear the full Arab burka often wear something more fitted when at home in private and amongst women. Choose clothes that will allow you to feel trimmer and you'll get a boost of energy.

In a nutshell, it's all about energy. Once you accept that you no longer have to hide yourself or your weight issue under clothing, a *psychological* weight will be lifted off your shoulders! There's a real boost of confidence to be had simply from a new garment or even a few inexpensive new accessories to brighten up your style and mood! In my husband's Indian culture, new clothing is always bought to celebrate festival days and New Year, because it injects a brand new feeling of energy and confidence to propel you forward!

Tell yourself you're going to dress confidently and that you'll feel like a slimmer person from now on, and before long you'll be on the way to actually *becoming* that person. That's when things 'become *effortless*', as coach Ali Campbell puts it.[2] As I said, the unconscious mind likes to justify itself!

So, in conclusion, get rid of all your 'fat' clothes and those which act as an excuse to overeat. As you lose weight, give them to charity, or to friends, or sell them on eBay. By ridding your wardrobe of your baggier clothes, you'll be cutting off all recourse to 'wiggle room', where excuses hide! Those who keep their 'fat' clothes aren't actually convinced that they'll keep the weight off. *But those who throw away their 'fat' clothes are throwing away their 'fat' self forever!'*

Lastly, having clothes that fit is a powerful incentive to eat right so as not to put any weight on again. Speaking for myself, my daily 'uniform' is jeans, so I own quite a few pairs of rather expensive 'skinny' designer jeans. Personally, I can't *afford* to put on weight ... can *you*?

Appendix I

The Health Benefits of Herbs and Spices

Here is a list of the health benefits of commonly used herbs and spices to assist you in harnessing their properties for yourself:

- *Basil:* Calms nervous irritability, has an analgesic effect on headaches. Not to be used in pregnancy.
- *Cayenne pepper, paprika and chilli powder:* Help curb hunger pangs and boost metabolic rate. Their main ingredient, capsaicin, increases satiety!
- *Cinnamon:* The antioxidant level (polyphenols) in cinnamon is greater than that in pomegranates and blueberries, per volume Cinnamon regulates blood sugar levels and fights inflammation. Use the pure, freshly ground cinnamon or cinnamon sticks (in stews for example), *not* the sugared kind.
- *Coriander:* Rich in iron, the seeds aid digestion and increase lactation in breastfeeding women.
- *Cumin seeds:* A good source of iron and magnesium; these aid digestion and provide relief from diarrhoea, nausea and flatulence. Detoxifying and anti-carcinogenic, they also boost immunity. Possibly effective against asthma and arthritis.
- *Dill:* A digestive and anti-flatulence aid.
- *Garlic:* A natural antibiotic. Strengthens the immune system, lowers cholesterol, reduces vulnerability to infection, improves circulation, helps to reduce high blood pressure, aids digestion. Anti-fungal, anti-bacterial, anti-inflammatory, antioxidant, anti-parasitic, detoxifying properties. Wild garlics ('ramsons') are good if you can find them.
- *Ginger:* Warming, circulation boosting, a digestive aid; helps to reduce nausea and to increase appetite in convalescents.
- *Horseradish:* Warming, helps reduce rheumatic conditions and fevers. Increases circulation, stimulates digestion, calms stomach cramps and wind. Don't consume industrial versions mixed with cream and sugar!

- *Lemon juice:* The vitamins A and C in lemons protect the nose, throat, mouth and lungs and have antiseptic properties. Lemon juice supports liver function, builds immunity and helps to increase a sense of vitality.
- *Onions and chives:* Stimulate digestion, increase nutrient absorption, prevent growth of harmful bacteria in digestive and urinary systems (anti-bacterial and antiseptic properties).
- *Oregano:* Anti-microbial and antioxidant.
- *Parsley:* An excellent source of vitamin A, vitamin C and vitamin K. A good source of iron and folate. It is high in folic acid, a cardiovascular protector. Its volatile oils and flavanoids are antioxidant and anti-inflammatory. It protects the immune system and studies suggest it could protect against some forms of rheumatoid arthritis. Note: Those with kidney or gallbladder problems might avoid parsley as it contains a substance called oxalates which could exacerbate the problem.
- *Pepper:* A digestive and anti-flatulence aid. Anti-inflammatory, anti-bacterial and antioxidant properties; stimulates absorption of micro-nutrients, provides relief from sinusitis and nasal congestion in Ayurvedic medicine (sucking a few peppercorns can provide relief from a dry cough and throat irritation).
- *Rosemary:* In moderation good for joint pain and poor circulation, but in excess raises blood pressure, so use with care.
- *Sage:* Its oil has anti-bacterial, anti-viral and anti-fungal properties. Said to strengthen the nervous system and improve alertness, sage is used in some European countries to treat stomach upsets.
- *Sesame seeds (black or white):* Rich in calcium. Sprinkle on salads, grilled meats or stir-fries, or mix into smoothies or yogurts.
- *Sunflower seeds:* Contain selenium, which helps fight cancer and heart disease and boosts the immune system. Good source of essential fatty acids, rich in vitamin E, amino acids and calcium, zinc, potassium and magnesium. Help to reduce cholesterol and are a good source of dietary fibre.
- *Thyme:* Soothes abdominal cramps and improves digestion.
- *Turmeric:* Recent research suggests that curcumin, the main ingredient, reduces heart enlargement, so lowering the risk of heart failure, and may help prevent Alzheimer's disease. Use half a teaspoon in cooking; can be added to vegetable dishes, stews and curries with other seasonings when the pan is hot, as it needs to be 'fried' to best effect.

Appendix II

'Super-foods'

The super-foods shown in *italics* are especially potent providers of vital nutrients which you should eat multiple times per week. For a very comprehensive list of super-foods – and the 'super-nutrients' they comprise – Dr Steven Pratt's very informative book *SuperHealth* is highly recommended. This list is by no means exhaustive!

Protein-rich Foods

Eggs
All *eggs*, though the duck egg is somewhat higher in fat.
Fish
cod, farmed oysters and clams, farmed rainbow trout, herring, *mackerel, sardines*, shrimp, *white tuna, wild salmon*
Milk Products
fromage frais, quark, yogurt: organic plain live cultured yogurt and kefir (non-sweetened liquid pouring yogurt)
Soy or Soya
Soy, or soya, is a powerful high-protein food. But it must be non-genetically modified (non-GM) and preferably organically produced. Children should avoid eating it too frequently and women who have suffered breast cancer should consult their medical professional regarding how much soy to eat, because it contains plant-based hormones called phyto-oestrogens. That said, it is a valuable source of plant-based omega-3 fatty acids and many vitamins and minerals and is an excellent alternative to animal protein (the only plant-based complete protein source). It has anti-carcinogenic and cholesterol-reducing and detoxifying qualities and is consumed as a daily staple in countries like Japan and Korea. It is important to ensure your iodine levels are sufficient if you consume soy regularly, so check your vitamin supplement or use iodized salt.
edamame (green soya beans), miso, soy milk, soy nuts, soy yoghurt, tofu
White Meat

skinless chicken, turkey
Pulses
All beans and pulses including chickpeas, green beans, green peas, kidney beans, lentils, pinto, string beans, sugar snap peas, etc.

Wholegrains

Amaranth, barley, brown rice, buckwheat, Bulgar wheat, cous-cous, ground flaxseed, linseed, millet, oat bran, oats, quinoa, rye, spelt, wheatgerm, wild rice

Vegetables, Fruits, Berries and Nuts

Green
apples, artichokes, *asparagus, avocado, broccoli, broccoli sprouts, Bok-Choi, Brussels sprouts, cabbage, collard greens*, green peas, green peppers, *kale, kiwi fruit, limes*, peas, pears, *romaine lettuce, seaweed, spinach*, string beans, sugar snap peas, *watercress*
Red
apples, goji berries, pink grapefruit, *plums, pomegranates, prunes, red cabbage, red grapes*, red peppers, strawberries, *tomatoes, watermelon* (high in a super-nutrient called glutathione)
White
cauliflower, chives, daikon (white radish), garlic, leeks, onions, spring onions (shallots)
coconut The coconut is actually a fruit, not a nut, and a rich source of medium-chain fatty acids (MCFAs) like lauric acid, which are not readily stored in the body but easily digested and used as energy. Organic fresh or freshly-packaged unsweetened coconut milk is the best way to take advantage of these properties, as dried coconut is high in fat and can turn rancid quickly.
Yellow/Orange
apricots, butternut squash, carrots, grapefruit, guava, mandarins, *orange and yellow peppers*, oranges, persimmons, pumpkins, sweet potatoes, tangerines
Dried Fruit (in moderation due to high sugar content)
apples, apricots, black raisins, *blueberries*, cherries, *cranberries*, figs, prunes (all of these no sugar added)
Berries

black and purples grapes, blackberries, blueberries, cherries, cranberries, goji berries, raspberries, strawberries, all other berries, blackcurrants, redcurrants
Nuts
almonds, cashew nuts, hazelnuts, *peanut butter,* pecans, *pistachios, pumpkin seeds, sesame seeds, sunflower seeds, walnuts*
Spices
aniseed, basil, black pepper, caraway seeds, cayenne pepper, chilli, cinnamon, cumin, curry powder, fennel seeds, ginger, nutmeg, oregano, rosemary, saffron, sage, thyme (and so on). (*See also Appendix I, page 000.*)

Extras
cinnamon, dark unprocessed honey, extra virgin olive oil, garlic, green tea, Oolong tea, *raw cocoa or cacao* (or dark 70 per cent plus chocolate), Roiboos tea

Notes and References

Introduction

1. Acknowledgements to Chris Howard of the Academy of Wealth and Achievement.
2. Acknowledgements to Steve Linder of www.sricoaching.com.
3. Ibid.
4. The Law of Requisite Variety: Ashby, W. R., 'Requisite Variety and its implications for the control of complex systems', Cybernetica 1 (1958), no.2

Chapter 1: Before You Start

1. Acknowledgements to Steve Linder of www.sricoaching.com.
2. The Oxford English Dictionary
3. http://www.allaboutlifechallenges.org/bulimia-and-anorexia-faq.htm; Beers, M. H., and Berkow, R. (eds), 'Eating Disorders: Anorexia nervosa' in The Merck Manual of Diagnosis and Therapy, 17th edition, Merck Research Laboratories, NJ, 1999); http://ezinearticles.com/?Bulimia-Side-Effects---The-Effects-of-Bulimia-on-Your-Health---Nurses-Guide&id=1693797; http://helpguide.org/mental/anorexia_signs_symptoms_causes_treatment.htm

Chapter 2: *28 Keys to Thinking Differently*

1. I'm quoting Chinese philosopher Lao-tzu (640–531 BC), not Confucius, as is commonly believed. Michael Moncur states that: 'Although this is the popular form of this quotation, a more correct translation from the original Chinese would be "The journey of a thousand miles begins beneath one's feet." Rather than emphasizing the first step, Lau Tzu regarded action as something that arose naturally from stillness. Another potential phrasing would be "Even the longest journey must begin where you stand."' http://www.quotationspage.com/quote/24004.html, 1 September 2004

2. Maxwell Maltz, MD, FICS, Psycho-cybernetics: A new way to get more living out of life, Wilshire Book Company/Prentice Hall, 1963; http://www.butler-bowdon.com/psychocybernets

3. D. O. Hebb, The Organization of Behaviour, Wiley & Sons, New York, 1949

4. Cabanac, M., Duclaux, R., and Spector, N. H., 'Sensory feedback in regulation of body weight: is there a ponderostat?', Nature 229 (1971), issue 5, 280, 125–7

5. http://www.historyguide.org/intellect/erasmus.html

6. Sarra Manning, 'The Truth about Downsizing', 'Stella' magazine, Sunday Telegraph, 23 January 2011, pp.34–9

7. 'Seventeen drafts, yes. I rise about at 5.30 in the morning. I write from six till eight, take a two-hour break, write from ten until twelve, take a two-hour break, write from two till four, take a two-hour break, write from six till eight, then it's bed by 9.30, sleep by 10 and up at 5.30 to do it again! The first draft probably took about eight weeks, i.e. probably 300 hours. The final version that you have there, the seventeenth draft, took 1,000 hours of work. I mention this because a lot of people, particularly young people, think that they're going to knock off a book this weekend. But it's damn hard work! And the only thing I'd say to those young people watching this show is when you've finished the first draft, you've only just about started.' Jeffery Archer interviewed by Amrita Tripathi, Jeffrey Archer on Books, Cricket and India, CNN-IBN, http://ibnlive.in.com/news/jeffrey-archer-on-books-cricket-and-india/66047-19.html

8. Acknowledgements to Steve Linder of www.sricoaching.com.

9. 'As habits are learned … cues in the environment become the triggers of predictable and automatic actions. When it comes to food, we are, in essence, following an eating script that has been written into the circuits of our brains.' David A. Kessler, MD, The End of Overeating: Taking control of the insatiable American appetite, Rodale Press, 2009, p.62

10. Keith Cunningham, www.keystothevault.com

11. J. P. Tangney and K. W. Fischer, Self-conscious Emotions: The psychology of shame, guilt, embarrassment, and pride, Guilford, New York, 1995

12. Thanks and gratitude to Steve Linder.

13. Harris R. Lieberman, PhD, 'Hydration and cognition: a critical review and recommendations for future research', Journal of the American College of Nutrition 26 (2007), no.90,005, 555S–61S

14. 'Increasing the variety of a food increases how much everyone eats. To demonstrate this, Dr. Barbara Rolls at Penn State has showed that if people are offered an assortment with three different flavours of yogurt, they're likely to consume an average of 23 percent more than if offered only one flavour… Most people know that all M&Ms taste alike. The colour is just added to the coating… The person with 10 colours [of M&Ms] will eat 43 more M&Ms (99 versus 56) than this friend with 7 colours. He does so because he thinks there's more variety, which increases how much he thinks he'll like the M&Ms…' Brian Wansink, PhD, Mindless Eating: Why we eat more than we think, Hay House, 2006, Chapter 3, references 17 and 21

15. Acknowledgements to Steve Linder.

16. The American author Napoleon Hill (26 October 1883–8 November 1970) was one of the earliest proponents of the Law of Attraction. This quotation comes from a talk about his meeting with Andrew Carnegie, once the richest man in the world and head of the Carnegie Steel Company, which was sold to J. P. Morgan in 1901 for $480 million. See Napoleon Hill, Think and Grow Rich, Combined Registry Company, Chicago, Illinois, 1937, p.14

17. Wakslak, C. J., and Trope, Y. , 'Cognitive consequences of affirming the self: the relationship between self-affirmation and object construal', Journal of Experimental Social Psychology 45 (2009), 927–32

18. For example, Koehn, S., Morris, T., and Watt, A. P., 'Efficacy of an imagery intervention to increase flow and performance', British Journal of Sports Medicine 11 (2006), no.1; www.stms. nl; http://en.wikipedia.org/wiki/Creative_visualization; Martin, Kathleen A., and Hall, Craig, R., 'Using mental imagery to enhance intrinsic motivation,' Journal of Sport and Exercise Psychology 17 (1995), issue 1

19. Cited in Robert Scaglione and William Cummins, Karate of Okinawa: Building Warrior Spirit, Tuttle Publishing, 1993

20. Quoting John Damascene, De Fide Orth., ii, 14

21. Koran 113:5

22. Ahmad.

23. Tirukkural, Verse 162

24. http://yoruba.unl.edu/yoruba.php-text=1c&view=2&uni=0&l=17.htm

25. http://www.bbc.co.uk/health/emotional_health/mental_health/disorders_munchausenssyndrome1.shtml

26. http://allpsych.com/journal/munchausen.html

27. http://en.wikipedia.org/wiki/Susan_Boyle

28. Ibid.

29. Hayes, Diane, and Ross, Catherine E., 'Body and mind: the effect of exercise, overweight, and physical health on psychological well-being', Journal of Health and Social Behaviour 27 (1986), 387–400

30. News release, CDC, Morbidity and Mortality Weekly Report 58, November 20, 2009

31. Statistics on obesity, physical activity and diet: England, 2011 (The Health and Social Care Information Centre), sections 2.2.1, 3.2 and table 7.12; http://www.ic.nhs.uk/webfiles/publications/003_Health_Lifestyles/opad11/Statistics_on_Obesity_Physical_Activity_and_Diet_England_2011_revised_Aug11.pdf

32. William J. Cromie, 'Meditation changes temperatures: mind controls body in extreme experiments', Harvard University Gazette, April 18, 2002

33. Ibid. (My italics.)

34. Richard Hoggart, introduction to D. H. Lawrence, Lady Chatterley's Lover, second edition, 1961, p.viii

35. David A. Kessler, MD, The End of Overeating: Taking control of the insatiable American appetite, Rodale Press, 2009, p.218

36. Eric Sabo, the NBC Digital Health Network; also cited in Robert Scaglione and William Cummins, Karate of Okinawa: Building warrior spirit, Tuttle Publishing, 1993

37. Robert T. Kiyosaki with Sharon L. Lechter, CPA, Rich Dad, Poor Dad: What the rich teach their kids – that you can learn too, Sphere, 2009, p.223

38. Kessler, op. cit., p.182

39. Ibid., p.183.

40. Quoted ibid, p.186.

41. http://ga.water.usgs.gov/edu/propertyyou.html

42. http://ga.water.usgs.gov/edu/propertyyou.html, quoting Dr Jeffrey Utz, paediatric neuroscientist at Allegheny University.

43. Lisa Conti, 'Artificial Sweeteners Confound the Brain; May Lead to Diet Disaster: Substances like Splenda trigger reward activity but do not satiate a sugar craving', http://www.scientificamerican.com/article.cfm?id=artificial-sweeteners-confound-the-brain, June 5, 2008

44. http://www.medicinenet.com/caffeine/page5.htm

45. Kessler, op. cit., p.85

46. 'Conditioning can happen quickly. In one study, people were given a high-sugar, high-fat snack for five consecutive mornings. For days afterward, they wanted something sweet at about the same time each morning that they had been fed the snack, even though they had not previously snacked at that time.' L. C. Haverkort and A. Prakken, MSc thesis, Wangeningen University, Netherlands, 1992, quoted in Kessler, op. cit., p.51

47. Doris Wild Helmering and Dianne Hales, Think Thin, Be Thin, Broadway Books, 2004, p.77, quoted in Brian Wansink, PhD, in Mindless Eating: Why we eat more than we think , Hay House 2010, Chapter 7, note 10

48. David A. Kessler, MD, The End of Overeating: Taking control of the insatiable American appetite, Rodale Press, 2009

49. See Richard J. Johnson, MD, Timothy Gower and Elizabeth Gollub, The Sugar Fix: The high fructose fallout that is making you fat and sick, Rodale Press, 2008

50. Edmund T. Rolls, 'The orbitofrontal cortex and reward', Oxford Journals/Life Sciences and Medicine/Cerebral Cortex 10 (2000), issue 3, 284–94

51. Helen Phillips, 'The Pleasure Seekers', New Scientist, 11 October 2003

52. Rolls, op. cit.

53. Fredrickson, B. L., Mancuso, R. A., Branigan, C., and Tugade, M. M., 'The undoing effect of positive emotions', Motivation and Emotion 24 (2000), 237–58

54. Thanks to Steve Linder of www.sricoaching.com for this concept and wording.

Chapter 3: *10 Super-Strategies*

1. '"Calorie restriction is pretty much the only thing out there that we know will not just prevent disease but also extend maximal life span," says Dr. Marc Hellerstein, a nutritionist at the University of California, Berkeley, who studies the biological effects of fasting.' Bryan Walsh, 'Eat Less, Live Longer?', www.time.com, Thursday, Feb. 11, 2010; Salk Institute, 'Eat Less, Live Longer? Gene links calorie restriction to longevity', Science Daily, 2 May 2007

2. Thanks for that idea to Richard Bandler, founder of NLP.

3. Quoted in Christopher Howard, Instant Wealth: Wake up rich, Wiley, 2010, pp.191–2

4. Wansink, Brian, and Cheney, Matthew M., 'Super bowls: serving bowl size and food consumption', Journal of the American Medical Association 293, no.14 (April 2005), 727–8

5. Chaput, Jean-Philippe, Després, Jean-Pierre, Bouchard, Claude, Tremblay, Angelo, 'The association between sleep duration and weight gain in adults: a 6-year prospective study from the Quebec Family Study', Sleep 31 (2008), no.4, 517–23

6. Columbia University's Mailman School of Public Health and the Obesity Research Center, Analysis of data taken from the National Health and Nutrition Examination Survey I (NHANES I), presented at the North American Association for the Study of Obesity (NAASO)'s Annual Scientific Meeting, Nov. 14–18, 2004.

7. Quoted in Mary Shomon, 'Lack of sleep may lead to excess weight: study finds link between hours of sleep and risk of obesity', About.com Guide, November 18, 2004, http://thyroid.about.com/b/2004/11/18/lack-of-sleep-may-lead-to-excess-weight-study-finds-link-between-hours-of-sleep-and-risk-of-obesity.htm

8. Quoted in Jeane Chapin, 'Lack of Sleep Linked to Obesity in National Studies, The Tiger, Jan. 21st, 2005, http://thetigernews.com/news.php?aid=2739&sid=#

9. Jennifer LaRue Huget, http://voices.washingtonpost.com/checkup/2010/04/how_do_unschoolers_learn_what.html

10. Lifschitz, Carlos H., 'Feeding problems in infants and children', Current Treatment Optios in Gastroenterology 4 (2001), no.5, 451–7; DOI: 10.1007/s11938-001-0010-x http://www.springerlink.com/content/g60553206362h910/

11. Gross, Lee S., Li Li, Ford, Earl S., and Liu, Simin, 'Increased consumption of refined carbohydrates and the epidemic of Type 2 diabetes in the United States: an ecologic assessment', American Journal of Clinical Nutrition 79 (2004), no.5, 774–9

12. See Richard J. Johnson, MD, Timothy Gower and Elizabeth Gollub, The Sugar Fix: The high-fructose fallout that is making you fat and sick, Rodale Press, 2008

13. Brian Wansink, PhD, Mindless Eating: Why we eat more than we think, Hay House Ltd, 2006, p.60

Chapter 4: *10 Powerful Food Habits*

1. For nutritional breakdown and nutrition rating estimates, www.caloriecount.about.com is a useful resource.

2. http://www.jamieoliver.com/jamies-ministry-of-food/

3. Veldhorst, M., et al., 'Protein-induced satiety: effects and mechanisms of different proteins', Physiolog. Behav. 94 (2008), 300–307; Westerterp-Plantenga, M. S., 'Protein intake and energy balance', Regul. Pept. 149 (2008), 67–9; Paddon-Jones, D., et al., 'Protein, weight management and satiety', American Journal of Clinical Nutrition 87 (suppl.) (2008), 1558S–61S

4. http://www.eurekalert.org/pub_releases/2010-11/uoc-drf112310.php
5. www.patrickholford.com
6. Thanks to Patrick Holford for introducing me to this fascinating concept in his excellent book Optimum Nutrition for your Child: How to boost your child's health, behaviour and IQ (Piatkus Books, 2008).
7. http://www.enotes.com/science-fact-finder/human-body/how-many-cells-human-body
8. In The End of Overeating: Taking control of the insatiable American appetite (Rodale Press, 2009), David A. Kessler, MD, writes: 'I've learned to recognize overeating in restaurants all over America. It's not hard, because people who have been conditioned to overeat behave distinctively. They attack their food with a special kind of gusto. I've seen them lift their forks, readying their next bite before they've swallowed the previous one, and I've watched as they reach across the table to spear a companion's French fries or the last morsel of someone else's dessert' (Introduction, p.xv).
9. Theravada meal chant, food requisite verse.
10. Birch, L. L., Deysher, M., 'Caloric compensation and sensory specific satiety: evidence for self-regulation of food intake by young children' Appetite 7 (1986), no.4, 323–31; http://www.ncbi.nlm.nih.gov/pubmed/3789709

Chapter 5: Be Nutritionally Aware and Exercise Savvy

1. Patrick Bradley, 'The ponderostat and a physiological model of obesity', The American Journal of Clinical Nutrition, http://www.ajcn.org/cgi/reprint/31/11/1975.
2. Rodin, Judith, Moskowitz, Howard R., Bray, George A., 'Taste responsiveness, weight loss, and the ponderostat', Physiol. Behav. 11(S) (1973), 641–5; Nisbett, R. E., Hanson Jr., L. R., Harris, A., and Stair, A., 'Relationship between obesity, weight loss and taste responsiveness', Physiology & Behavior 17 (1976), issue 4, pp.591–7
3. Sonia Nigro Rosso, 'Which Diet or Dietary Approach – A Consumer's Approach?' in Progress in Obesity Research 9, eds Geraldo Medeiros-Neto, Alfredo Halpern and Claude Bouchard, Chapter 191

4. Stephen Pratt, MD, with Sharyn Kolberg, SuperHealth, Dutton Books, 2008

5. Ibid.

6. Lustig, R. H., 'The Fructose Epidemic', The Bariatrician, June 2009

7. Pinckney, E. R. and C., The Cholesterol Controversy, Sherbourne Press, Los Angeles, 1973, pp.127–31

8. http://en.wikipedia.org/wiki/Butylated_hydroxyanisole

9. http://en.wikipedia.org/wiki/Butylated_hydroxytoluene

10. David A. Kessler, MD, The End of Overeating: Taking control of the insatiable American appetite, Rodale Press, 2009, pp.141–3

11. Johnson, R. J., Segal, M. S., Sautin, Y., Nakagawa, T., Feig, D. I., Kang, D-H., Gersch, M. S., Benner, S., and Sánchez-Lozada, L., 'Potential role of sugar (fructose) in the epidemic of hypertension, obesity and the metabolic syndrome, diabetes, kidney disease, and cardiovascular disease', American Journal of Clinical Nutrition 86 (2007); http:/www.ajcn.org/content/86/4/899.abstract

12. Richard J. Johnson, MD, Timothy Gower and Elizabeth Gollub, The Sugar Fix: The high fructose fallout that is making you fat and sick, Rodale Press, 2008, p.53

13. Peter J. Havel, PhD, et al., 'Dietary fructose: implications for dysregulation of energy homeostasis and lipid/carbohydrate metabolism', Nutrition Reviews 63 (2005), quoted ibid., p.66.

14. Beck-Nielsen, H., Pedersen, O., Lindskov, H. O., 'Impaired cellular insulin binding and insulin sensitivity induced by high-fructose feeding in normal subjects', American Journal of Clinical Nutrition 33 (1980), 273–8, quoted ibid.

15. Havel, Peter. J., op. cit., 133–47, quoted ibid., p.111

16. 'Eat any sugar alcohol lately?', Yale-New Haven Hospital, 3 October 2005; http://www.ynhh.org/about-us/sugar_alcohol.aspx?source=sugar_alcohol.html.

17. Just, T., Pau, H. W., Engel, U., Hummel, T., 'Cephalic phase insulin release in healthy humans after taste stimulation?', Appetite 51 (2008), no.3, 622–7; Rohner-Jeanrenaud, F., Proietto, J., Rivest, R. W., and Jeanrenaud, B., 'Taste-induced changes in plasma insulin and glucose turnover in lean and genetically obese rats', Diabetes 37 (1988), no.6, 773–9, http://

diabetes.diabetesjournals.org/content/37/6/773; Berthoud, H. R., Trimble, E. R., Siegel, E. G., Bereiter, D. A., and Jeanrenaud, B., 'Cephalic-phase insulin secretion in normal and pancreatic islet-transplanted rats', American Journal of Physiology-Endocrinology and Metabolism 238 (1980), no.4, E336–40

18. Magnuson, B. A., Burdock, G. A., Doull, J., et al., 'Aspartame: a safety evaluation based on current use levels, regulations, and toxicological and epidemiological studies', Critical Reviews in Toxicology 37 (2007), no.8, 629–727

19. Ferland, A., Brassard, P., Poirier, P., 'Is aspartame really safer in reducing the risk of hypoglycemia during exercise in patients with Type 2 diabetes?', Diabetes Care 30, no.7 (2007), http://care.diabetesjournals.org/content/30/7/e59

20. Taken from: http://www.fitnessandpower.com/training/cardio/150-pha-training-workout

Afterword

1. 'The Prison Pounds Mystery', as reported by Brian Wansink, PhD, in Mindless Eating: Why we eat more than we think, Hay House, 2010, pp.40–41

2. Ali Campbell, Just Get On With It! A caring, compassionate kick up the ass!, Hay House, 2010

Resources

Books

Elana Amsterdam, *The Gluten-Free Almond Flour Cookbook*, Celestial Arts, 2009

Richard Bandler and John Grinder, *Frogs into Princes: Introduction to Neurolinguistic Programming*, Eden Grove Editions, 1979

Ross Bridgeford, *The Alkaline Diet Recipe Book*; http://www.energiseforlife.com

Ali Campbell, *Just Get On With It! A caring, compassionate kick up the ass!*, Hay House, 2010

Alan Carr, *The Easy Way to Stop Smoking*, Allen Carr, 1985

Roni deLuz, *21 Pounds in 21 Days: The Martha's Vineyard diet detox*, HarperCollins, 2007

Rocco Dispirito, *Now Eat This!*, Ballantine Books, 2010

Audrey Eyton, *The 'F' Plan*, Book Club Associates, 1982

Helen Foster, *The Easy GI Diet: Use the glycaemic index to lose weight and gain energy*, Hamlyn, 2004

GI: How to succeed using a glycaemic index diet, Collins Gem, HarperCollinsPublishers, 2005

GI: Lose weight for good and enjoy your food, Collins Gem, HarperCollinsPublishers, 2006

D. O. Hebb, *The Organization of Behaviour*, Wiley & Sons, New York, 1949

Napoleon Hill, *Think and Grow Rich*, Fawcett Books, 1975

Patrick Holford, *The Optimum Nutrition Bible: The book you have to read if you care about your health*, Piatkus Books, 2004

—,*Optimum Nutrition for your Child: How to boost your child's health, behaviour and IQ*, Piatkus Books, 2008

Christopher Howard, *Instant Wealth – Wake Up Rich!: Discover the secret of the new entrepreneurial mind*, John Wiley & Sons, 2010

Susan Jeffers, *Feel the Fear and Do It Anyway*, Century, 1988

Richard J. Johnson, MD, Timothy Gower and Elizabeth Gollub, *The Sugar Fix: The high fructose fallout that is making you fat and sick*, Rodale Press, 2008

David A. Kessler, MD, *The End of Overeating: Taking control of the insatiable American appetite*, Rodale Press, 2009

Robert Kiyosaki, Rich Dad, *Poor Dad 2 – Cash Flow Quadrant: Rich Dad's guide to financial freedom*, Warner Books in associations with CASHFLOW Technologies, Inc., 2000

Paul McKenna, *Instant Confidence*, Bantam Press, 2006

—, *I Can Make You Thin: 90 day success journal*, Bantam Press, 2007

Maxwell Maltz, MD, FICS, *Psycho-cybernetics: A new way to get more living out of life*, Wilshire Book Company/Prentice Hall, 1963

Jamie Oliver, *Cook with Jamie: My guide to making you a better cook*, Michael Joseph, 2006

—, *Jamie's Ministry of Food: Anyone can learn to cook in 24 hours*, Michael Joseph, 2008

Steven Pratt, MD, with Sharyn Kolberg, *SuperHealth: 10 Simple Steps, 6 Easy Weeks, 1 Longer, Healthier Life*, Dutton Books, 2008

—, with Kathy Matthews, *SuperFoodsRx: Fourteen foods that will change your life*, William Morrow & Co., 2004

Anthony Robbins, *Unlimited Power*, HarperCollins, 1987

Matt Roberts, *The PHA Workout: A revolutionary new system to halve your workout time*, Dorling Kindersley, 2005

J. P. Tangney and K. W. Fischer, *Self-conscious Emotions: The psychology of shame, guilt, embarrassment, and pride*, Guilford, 1995

Brian Wansink, PhD, *Mindless Eating: Why we eat more than we think*, Hay House, 2010

Nick Williams, *Unconditional Success: Loving the work we were born to do*, Bantam Press, 2002

Anthony Worrall Thompson, with Dr Mabel Blades and Jane Suthering, *Anthony Worrall Thompson's GI Diet*, Kyle Cathie Ltd, 2005

Websites

www.anniemation.co.uk
Annie will be able to help you with a more beautiful and balanced living environment while you are optimizing your health and body image!

www.alicampbell.com
Ali Campbell is one of the UK's foremost NLP experts and gave me advice and moral support when I most needed it.

www.anorexiabulimiacare.org.uk
Please seek help if you believe you may have an eating disorder, before it is too late.

www.aqualibria.com
The UK's premier hydrotherapy clinic on Harley Street.

www.becomealifestyler.com
One of Designer Health Centers' cutting-edge nutritional and lifestyle programmes.

www.caloriecountabout.com
Useful calorie counting website.

www.designerhealthcenters.com
For Dr Isaac Jones, wellness and weight-loss expert with global reach.

www.glycemicindex.com and www.gilisting.com
Useful websites for checking out the glycaemic index of foods.

www.raystevensfitnessclubs.co.uk
Olympic medallist Ray Steven's programmes for fitness and martial arts.

www.sricooaching.com and www.sriuniversity.com
Cutting-edge NLP Neurostrategy training.

www.thefooddoctor.com
Optimum nutritional programs, advice and products.

To contact Natasha Reddy and find out more about the New Health Model movement, email **support@designerhealthcenters.com** and reference Natasha Reddy and this book.